WP 18 SLA
9AS137

withdrawn 97
03/19.

1/18 2/13

D0315477

HINCHINBROOKE

Key Questions
OBSTETRICS AND
GYNAECOLOGY

Key Questions in
OBSTETRICS AND
GYNAECOLOGY

R.J. Slade
FRCS (Glas), MRCOG
Senior Registrar in Obstetrics and Gynaecology,
University Hospital of Wales,
Cardiff, UK

E. Laird
MRCOG, MRNZCOG
Senior Registrar in Obstetrics and Gynaecology,
Northampton General Hospital,
Northampton, UK

G. Beynon
FRCS (Ed), MRCOG
Senior Registrar in Obstetrics and Gynaecology,
Princess Anne Hospital,
Southampton, UK

© BIOS Scientific Publishers Limited, 1994

First published 1994

All rights reserved. No part of this book may be reproduced or transmitted, in any form or by any means, without permission.

A CIP catalogue record for this book is available from the British Library.

ISBN 1 872748 73 2

BIOS Scientific Publishers Ltd
St Thomas House, Becket Street, Oxford OX1 1SJ, UK
Tel. +44 (0)865 726286. Fax +44 (0)865 246823

DISTRIBUTORS

Australia and New Zealand
DA Information Services
648 Whitehorse Road, Mitcham
Victoria 3132

India
Viva Books Private Limited
4346/4C Ansari Road
New Delhi 110 002

Singapore and South East Asia
Toppan Company (S) PTE Ltd
38 Liu Fang Road, Jurong
Singapore 2262

USA and Canada
Books International Inc.
PO Box 605, Herndon, VA 22070

Typeset by Herb Bowes Graphics, Oxford, UK.
Printed by Information Press Ltd, Eynsham, UK.

CONTENTS

ABBREVIATIONS

A	Androstenedione
AC	Abdominal circumference
ACTH	Adrenocorticotrophic hormone
AFP	Alpha fetoprotein
AFV	Amniotic fluid volume
AID	Artificial insemination by donor
AIDS	Acquired immune deficiency syndrome
AIH	Artificial insemination by husband
AP	Anteroposterior
APH	Antepartum haemorrhage
ARDS	Adult respiratory distress syndrome
ARM	Artificial rupture of the membranes
BD	Two times per day *(bis in die)*
BP	Blood pressure
BPD	Biparietal diameter
bpm	Beats per minute
BPP	Biophysical profile
cAMP	Cyclic adenyl monophosphate
CIN	Cervical intraepithelial neoplasia
cm/h	Centimetres per hour
CPD	Cephalopelvic disproportion
CPR	Cardiopulmonary resuscitation
CRL	Crown–rump length
CSF	Cerebrospinal fluid
CT	Computerized tomography
CTG	Cardiotocograph
CVS	Chorionic villus sampling
CXR	Chest X-ray
D&C	Dilatation and curettage
DDAVP	Vasopressin
DHEA	Dehydroepiandrosterone
DHEAS	Dehydroepiandrosterone sulphate
DIC	Disseminated intravascular coagulation
DM	Diabetes mellitus
DNA	Deoxyribonucleic acid
DUB	Dysfunctional uterine bleeding
DVT	Deep vein thrombosis
ECG	Electrocardiogram
ECV	External cephalic version
ELISA	Enzyme-linked immunosorbent assay
ELP	Erect lateral pelvimetry

EMG	Electromyography
ERPOC	Evacuation of retained products of conception
ESR	Erythrocyte sedimentation rate
EUA	Examination under anaesthetic
FBC	Full blood count
FDP	Fibrin degradation products
FIGO	International Federation of Gynaecologists and Obstetricians
FSH	Follicle stimulating hormone
g	Grams
g/dl	Grams per decilitre
GA	General anaesthetic
GFR	Glomerular filtration rate
GIFT	Gamete intrafallopian transfer
GIT	Gastrointestinal tract
GnRH	Gonadotrophin releasing hormone
GP	General practitioner
G6PD	Glucose-6-phosphate dehydrogenase
GSI	Genuine stress incontinence
GSV	Gestational sac volume
GTT	Glucose tolerance test
HbF	Fetal haemoglobin
HC	Head circumference
hCG	Human chorionic gonadotrophin
HDL	High density lipoproteins
HIV	Human immunodeficiency virus
HLA	Human leukocyte antigens
hMG	Human menopausal gonadotrophin
HPL	Human placental lactogen
HPV	Human papilloma virus
HRT	Hormone replacement therapy
HSV	Herpes simplex virus
HWY	Hundred women years
IBS	Irritable bowel syndrome
IgG	Immunoglobulin G
IgM	Immunoglobulin M
IM	Intramuscular
IOL	Induction of labour
IPI	Intraperitoneal insemination
ITP	Idiopathic thrombocytopenic purpura
ITU	Intensive therapy unit
IU	International units
IUCD	Intrauterine contraceptive device
IUD	Intrauterine death
IUGR	Intrauterine growth retardation
IUI	Intrauterine insemination

IV	Intravenous
IVC	Inferior vena cava
IVF	*In vitro* fertilization
IVP	Intravenous pyelogram
IVU	Intravenous urogram
kcal	Kilocalories
kg	Kilograms
l/min	Litres per minute
LA	Local anaesthetic
LDL	Low density lipoproteins
LFT	Liver function tests
LH	Luteinizing hormone
LHRH	Luteinizing hormone releasing hormone
LLETZ	Large loop excision of the transformation zone
LSCS	Lower segment Caesarean section
mg	Milligrams
MHC	Major histocompatibility complex
MIS	Minimally invasive surgery
ml/min	Millilitres per minute
mmHg	Millimetres of mercury
mmol	Millimoles
mmol/l	Millimoles per litre
μmol/l	Micromoles per litre
MoM	Multiples of the median
mosmol	Milliosmoles
MPE	Maximum permitted exposure
MRI	Magnetic resonance imaging
MSSU	Midstream specimen of urine
NCEPOD	National Confidential Enquiry into Perioperative Death
NTD	Neural tube defect
OA	Occipito-anterior
OCP	Oral contraceptive pill
OD	Optical density
PCOS	Polycystic ovary syndrome
PCR	Polymerase chain reaction
PCT	Postcoital test
PE	Pulmonary embolus
PET	Pre-eclamptic toxaemia
PG	Prostaglandin
PGE	Prostaglandin E
PGF	Prostaglandin F
PID	Pelvic inflammatory disease
PIF	Prolactin inhibitory factor

PMS	Premenstrual syndrome
PO	By mouth *(per os)*
POD	Pouch of Douglas
POP	Progesterone only pill
PPH	Postpartum haemorrhage
PRF	Prolactin releasing factor
prn	As necessary *(pro re nata)*
PROM	Premature rupture of membranes
PTTK	Partial thromboplastin and kaolin time
QDS	Four times per day *(quater in die)*
RAMP	Rapid action matrix pregnancy test
RDS	Respiratory distress syndrome
RNA	Ribonucleic acid
RPOC	Retained products of conception
RSA	Recurrent spontaneous abortion
SC	Subcutaneous
SHBG	Sex hormone binding globulin
SL	Sublingual
SLE	Systemic lupus erythematosus
SR	Slow retard
SROM	Spontaneous rupture of membranes
SVC	Superior vena cava
T	Testosterone
TB	Tuberculosis
TBG	Thyroid binding globulin
TCRE	Transcervical resection of the endometrium
TDS	Three times per day *(ter in die)*
TENS	Transcutaneous electrical nerve stimulation
TFT	Thyroid function tests
TOP	Termination of pregnancy
TPHA	*Treponema pallidum* haemagglutination assay
TRH	Thyrotrophin releasing hormone
TSH	Thyroid stimulating hormone
TURP	Transurethral resection of the prostate
U&E	Urea and electrolytes
UPSI	Unprotected sexual intercourse
USS	Ultrasound scan
UTI	Urinary tract infection
V-V	Vesico-vaginal
VDRL	Venereal Disease Reference Laboratory
VIN	Vulval intraepithelial neoplasia
VLBW	Very low birthweight
VLDL	Very low density lipoproteins

VMA	Vanillyl mandelic acid
WCC	White cell count
WHO	World Health Organisation
ZIFT	Zygote intrafallopian transfer

PREFACE

In common with most postgraduate examinations, multiple choice questions are included in the Part II MRCOG examination.

This text comprises 360 multiple choice questions divided into six 'papers' of 60 questions each. The first three papers are obstetric in orientation and the next three gynaecological. This reflects the current arrangements in the Membership exam: in the morning candidates are presented with 60 MCQs followed by two obstetric essays; in the afternoon the same form applies for the gynaecological section. Each MCQ 'paper' should be completed within 1 hour.

Answers to the questions are provided at the back of the book, with brief explanations where needed. The reader is referred to the appropriate pages in *Key Topics in Obstetrics and Gynaecology* for a background to the question and its answer, and in some cases to supplementary references.

We have tried to ensure that the questions are not ambiguous but if you feel that any are, please let us know.

Finally it is important to realise that the examiners are not trying to trick you; take each question at face value and do not look for the catch. We hope that these questions and answers will help and encourage all those preparing for the exam.

Richard J. Slade
Euan Laird
Gareth Beynon

PRACTICE PAPER ONE

Allow 1 hour for the completion of all 60 questions

Answers are on p. 97

1.1   Amniotic fluid embolus

A   incidence of approximately 3 per million pregnancies
B   mortality rate of over 80%
C   more common in the first pregnancy
D   must be suspected in all cases of sudden maternal collapse
E   occurs before membrane rupture

1.2   The thyroid gland

A   in pregnancy increases in size as a result of the increase in thyroid blood flow and follicular hyperplasia
B   in pregnancy produces a rise in total thyroid hormone (T4) levels and a fall in triiodothyronine (T3) and thyroid binding globulin (TBG) levels
C   is a median thickening of endoderm in the floor of the pharynx between the third and fourth pharyngeal pouches
D   can be stimulated by placentally derived thyroid-like stimulating substances
E   is active in fetal lung maturation as thyroid hormones are required to initiate type II pneumocyte function

1.3   Puerperal psychosis

A   the patient may give a history of premenstrual syndrome
B   antidepressant drugs should be avoided in breast-feeding mothers
C   rejection of the baby is an early symptom
D   young mothers are a high-risk group
E   depressive feelings are reported in 50% of mothers

1.4   Analgesia in labour

A   TENS works by electrodes placed over the posterior rami of T4–T8
B   Entonox is a 60:40 mix of oxygen and nitrous oxide
C   pethidine has a metabolite which has convulsant properties
D   pethidine reduces pain scores by over 50%
E   the major side-effect of pethidine is to increase gastric emptying

1.5 The Report on Confidential Enquiries into Maternal Deaths in the United Kingdom

A analyses all maternal deaths, which are defined as any death of a woman in pregnancy and up to one year postnatally

B includes fortuitous deaths, which are deaths resulting from pre-existing disease or disease that developed during the pregnancy and which was aggravated by the pregnancy

C in the 1988–1990 Triennium, lists thromboembolic disease, hypertensive disorders of pregnancy, early pregnancy deaths, haemorrhage and amniotic fluid embolism as the five most common causes of direct maternal death

D is second only to The National Confidential Enquiries in Perioperative Death (NCEPOD) as the longest series of continuous clinical audit in the world

E for the Triennium 1988–1990, reports a mortality rate of approximately 10 deaths per 100 000 maternities

1.6 Episiotomy

A chromic catgut is the suture material of choice for repair

B inexact apposition of tissues may lead to dyspareunia

C subcuticular skin suturing is recommended to minimise late discomfort

D spontaneous tearing is to be preferred in a normal vaginal delivery

E extension to a third-degree tear may rarely result in colostomy formation

1.7 Antepartum haemorrhage

A defined as blood loss greater than 30 ml

B the frequency of placenta praevia is over 1%

C placenta praevia is associated with a previous Caesarean section

D placental abruption can recur in approximately 6%

E placental abruption is associated with presence of the lupus anticoagulant

1.8 The cervix uteri in pregnancy

A is 2 cm long in a nulliparous woman

B has biomechanical properties determined mainly by the connective tissue component rather than the smooth muscle component

C has a collagen content 25% less than the non-pregnant state

D when treated with PGE2 or PGF2 shows accelerated ripening

E may be aided in ripening by the cytokines, interleukin-1 and tumour necrosis factor

1.9 Presentations and positions of the fetus

A in face presentations mentoposterior position is compatible with vaginal delivery
B Kielland's rotational forceps should never be applied to a brow presentation
C in normal labour the sinciput is the denominator
D deep transverse arrest invariably results in operative delivery
E a transverse lie with the fetal back under the lower segment may present difficulties with delivery at Caesarean section

1.10 The following are involved in the biophysical profile

A fetal breathing movements
B fetal growth
C amniotic fluid volume
D a cardiotocograph
E umbilical cord Doppler

1.11 In prenatal diagnosis

A the most common indication for a fetal karyotype is advanced maternal age
B after a previously affected child, the risk of the next pregnancy having an abnormal fetal karyotype is 2.7%, if CVS is used for diagnosis
C 10% of all newborn Down's syndrome cases are due to a translocation trisomy
D Turner's syndrome-affected pregnant women should be offered termination of pregnancy because of the subsequent mental retardation
E in the Fragile [X] [q 27, 3] syndrome, 30% of the females show mental impairment

1.12 Antibiotics in pregnancy

A neonatal haemolysis is a side-effect of sulphonamides
B prophylaxis against beta-haemolytic streptococci is indicated if premature rupture of the membranes is to be treated conservatively
C the administration of recently introduced antibiotics without a proven safety record is justified in life-threatening infections
D folate antagonists may be administered in mid-trimester
E metronidazole is the drug of choice if anaerobic infection is suspected

1.13 Breech presentation

A occurs in 25% of cases at 32 weeks gestation
B an extended breech occurs in approximately 65% of cases
C cornual implantation of the placenta is an important cause
D at term less than 3% of pregnancies present by the breech
E the bitrochanteric diameter is greater than the biparietal diameter

1.14 A woman with a renal transplant

A has a greater than 50% chance of developing pre-eclampsia
B should come off azathioprine in the first trimester as it is very teratogenic
C can be safely delivered vaginally
D has a 100-fold risk of developing a gynaecological malignancy
E has a baby at risk of neonatal lymphocyte chromosomal aberrations

1.15 Rhesus disease

A the rhesus antigen is located on chromosome 6
B of the rhesus genes, C is the most clinically relevant
C cordocentesis is the standard procedure in estimating the degree of fetal haemolysis
D after 26 weeks gestation intrauterine transfusion should be considered if the fetal haematocrit is less than 30%
E irradiation of blood for intrauterine transfusion is contraindicated due to later adverse effects on the neonate

1.16 Cephalopelvic disproportion

A is defined as the failure of the fetal head to pass through the pelvis safely
B formation of the pelvis is dependent on vitamin C and phosphorus
C is more common in immigrant Asian patients in the UK
D can result in uterine rupture
E is a common cause of vesicovaginal fistula in the Third World

1.17 The fetal skull

A is in two parts during its development; the neurocranium and the somatocranium

B forms a posterior diamond-shaped fontanelle due to the junction of the midline sagittal sutures and the oblique lambdoid sutures

C has a relatively undeveloped mastoid, leaving the facial nerve particularly prone to damage during forceps deliveries

D has a biparietal diameter at term of 10.5 cm

E has an occipitofrontal diameter of 11.5 cm at term

1.18 Multiple pregnancy

A the degree of anaemia increases with multiple pregnancy, mainly as a consequence of increased plasma volume

B older mothers are less likely to conceive multiple pregnancies spontaneously

C prophylactic beta-adrenergic drugs are recommended in twin pregnancy due to the increased risk of premature labour

D there is a significant increase in the incidence of antepartum haemorrhage

E a significant delay of 5 minutes after the birth of the first triplet increases the risk for the second and third in terms of perinatal mortality

1.19 Development of the urinary system

A the kidney develops from the metanephros

B the trigone is endodermal in origin

C the mesonephric ducts will form the ureters

D the caudal end of the mesonephric duct can persist as Gartner's duct

E the bladder develops from the anterior portion of the cloaca

1.20 In the mother

A the ECG changes in pregnancy include T wave inversion in III, ST segment changes and Q waves

B Eisenmenger's syndrome has a 10% mortality in association with termination of pregnancy

C breast-feeding is contraindicated if she has heart failure treated with digoxin, as digoxin is toxic to the neonate and infant

D with a history of rheumatic heart disease and a penicillin allergy, vancomycin is the drug of choice at delivery

E with an artificial heart valve, warfarin is the anticoagulant of choice throughout the pregnancy

1.21 Regarding monitoring in labour

A external cardiotocography should be used continually in low-risk labour
B cardiotocography is an accurate method of predicting fetal hypoxia
C the use of an intrauterine pressure transducer may allow maximum recommended doses of Syntocinon to be exceeded
D a fall in the pH value of a fetal capillary blood sample of 0.016 U/h is acceptable during the first stage of normal labour
E any factor that converts labour from low to high risk is an indication for a fetal blood sample to measure pH

1.22 Epilepsy

A associated with a 1:40 risk of passing on to the sibling
B drug of choice is carbamazepine
C increased risk of placenta praevia
D increased risk of pre-eclampsia
E increase in operative deliveries

1.23 Diabetes in pregnancy

A diabetes may develop owing to the anti-insulin effects of pregnancy-related hormones such as HPL and cortisol
B maternal glucose crosses the placenta into the fetal circulation via active transport mechanisms
C a fasting blood glucose of greater than 8 mmol/l in a woman with hunger, polyuria and polydipsia is diagnostic of diabetes
D a glycosylated HbA_{1C} of greater than 6% is diagnostic of diabetes
E the administration of a standard WHO GTT of 100 g of oral glucose, after an overnight fast, may confirm the diagnosis of diabetes

1.24 Caesarean section

A the rate should ideally be less than 15%
B a Pfannenstiel incision is indicative of a lower segment operation when the patient has had a previous section
C a history of cephalopelvic disproportion is an absolute indication for elective section in a subsequent pregnancy
D the classical approach to the uterus is used when speed is important
E vertical incision over the lower uterus is known as the De Lee incision

1.25 Prerequisites for a forceps delivery

A a fully dilated cervix
B a relaxed uterus
C adequate analgesia
D catheterised bladder
E no cephalopelvic disproportion

1.26 Home confinement

A has recently begun to increase because of rises in obstetric intervention and an increase in the number of maternity support groups actively promoting home birth
B is associated with decreased rates of analgesia and episiotomy and increased rates of breast feeding and maternal satisfaction
C is specifically addressed in the Report of the Expert Maternity Group entitled 'Changing Childbirth'
D when it is unplanned is associated with a perinatal mortality rate considerably in excess of the normal UK perinatal mortality rate of 8/1000 total births
E was associated with two maternal deaths in the 1988–1990 Triennium reported by the Confidential Enquiries into Maternal Deaths in the United Kingdom

1.27 Infection in pregnancy

A hormonal changes in pregnancy predispose to a high incidence of vaginal candidiasis of the order of 16%
B transplacental infection with *Neisseria gonorrhoea* may lead to ophthalmia neonatorum
C rubella is the commonest congenital infection in the UK
D meconium staining of the liquor in premature labour is suggestive of toxoplasmosis
E varicella zoster infection is associated with greater degrees of neonatal morbidity if infection occurs just prior to delivery

1.28 The following statements concern shoulder dystocia

A the dystocia results due to the biacromial diameter failing to rotate
B associated with diabetic mothers
C a symphysiotomy is contraindicated
D suprapubic pressure is necessary to enable delivery of the anterior shoulder
E fracture of the clavicle can occur during delivery

1.29   In the immunology of pregnancy

A there are altered maternal antibody responses, the so-called 'blocking antibodies', which influence the maternal humoral immunity to the fetus
B Class I-like MHC antigens on extravillous cytotrophoblasts function to provide monitoring of tissue at risk of viral infection
C there is a 25% incidence of positive Anti-Ro (SS) antibodies in a woman with SLE
D the placenta may function in the rejection of the pregnancy due to its Class II MHC (HLA transplantation) antigens
E a woman with ITP carries no risk to her fetus as the IgG autoantibodies involved cannot cross the placenta

1.30   In normal labour

A effacement of the cervix is one important criterion for the onset of labour
B the cervicogram is the pivotal feature of the partogram
C crowning of the head occurs as the occipitoposterior diameter of the fetal skull reaches the introitus
D for active management of the third stage an oxytocic agent is given with delivery of the fetal head
E physiological management of the third stage is less likely to lead to a retained placenta

1.31   The following can be associated with hydrops fetalis

A trisomy 21
B parvovirus infection
C umbilical vein thrombosis
D 30% of cases are idiopathic
E G6PD deficiency

1.32   After delivery

A neonatal assessment using Apgar scores involves five neonatal parameters, namely respiration, heart rate, colour, reflex grasping and muscle tone   F
B if intubated, a neonate requires ventilation at a rate of 30–40/min, each for one second at a pressure of less than 30 cmH$_2$O   f   T
C a serum bilirubin of greater than 85 µmol/l is relatively common in a neonate   T
D kernicterus may occur in a neonate with a prolonged serum bilirubin of greater than 300 µmol/l   f   340µmol/l.
E tachypnoea, grunting and intercostal recession by the age of 4 hours are all necessary in the diagnosis of RDS in a neonate   F

1.33 Uterine activity in labour

A a pressure of 2000 kPa/15 min is generally regarded as hypertonic
B uterine activity is inhibited by adrenaline
C correcting a supine position may reverse uterine hypotonicity
D hypotonic activity is commoner in the multiparous
E neural stimulation is the prime force in uterine contractility

1.34 The diagnosis of intrauterine death can be confirmed by

A absence of fetal heart sounds
B absence of fetal movements
C Spalding's sign
D Robert's sign
E empty fetal bladder on USS

1.35 In a normal singleton pregnancy

A the average maternal weight gain is 14 kg, the gain being at a constant rate throughout the pregnancy
B a woman will require an extra daily calorific intake of 200–300 kcal after 36 weeks
C a woman may express colostrum in the second trimester
D oedema is ubiquitous secondary to renal retention of sodium due to an activated renin–angiotensin–aldosterone cascade
E the decrease in blood volume is at a maximum at 36 weeks

1.36 In anaemia related to pregnancy

A if serum ferritin levels are estimated then more than 80% of pregnant women are iron deficient in pregnancy
B inorganic ferric iron is most efficiently absorbed via the gastrointestinal tract
C fetal iron requirements are maximal at 32 weeks gestation
D megaloblastic anaemia is more likely due to folate than vitamin B12 deficiency
E a folate-deficient diet also predisposes to neural tube defects

1.37 Intrauterine growth retardation is associated with

A pre-eclampsia
B multigravidae
C placenta praevia
D a raised AFP
E twins

1.38 In pre-eclampsia

A 20% of all primigravidae are affected
B there are associations with short stature and Raynaud's disease
C the diagnosis can only be made greater than 20 weeks
D hypertension is defined as greater than 140/90 mmHg and proteinuria as greater than 500 mg/24 h
E a weight gain of greater than 2 kg/week is not significant

1.39 Cancer in pregnancy

A cancer affects 1 in 20 000 pregnancies
B a vaginal delivery may be feasible if cancer of the cervix is diagnosed in late pregnancy
C a vaginal delivery may be feasible if cancer of the vulva is diagnosed in late pregnancy
D carcinoma of the ovary is adversely affected by pregnancy in terms of survival
E vaginal delivery may occur after radical surgery for vulval cancer

1.40 Polyhydramnios is associated with

A premature labour
B cord prolapse
C postpartum haemorrhage
D Potter's syndrome
E trisomy 18

1.41 Prolonged pregnancy

A is defined by WHO as a pregnancy lasting 42 completed weeks or more and it is synonymous with postmaturity

B is associated with anencephaly

C may lead to shoulder dystocia as in 25% of prolonged pregnancies the fetus weighs 4000 g or more

D is more common in the summer and in those women with a positive personal and family history of prolonged pregnancy

E has a frequency of 10% when the dates are certain and 25% when the dates are uncertain

1.42 The coagulation system in pregnancy

A there is a rise in the platelet concentration

B clotting factor concentration increases, notably factors III and VI

C plasminogen activator is found in significant concentration in the placenta

D net changes result in a tendency to thromboembolism formation; a six-fold increased risk

E fibrin replaces elastic and muscle tissue in placental vessel walls, resulting in decreased blood flow

1.43 Postpartum haemorrhage is associated with

A retained products

B postmaturity

C multiple pregnancy

D primigravidae

E antepartum haemorrhage

1.44 In the puerperium

A the physiological hypercoagulable state of pregnancy lasts about 7 weeks, which has implications for the duration of thromboembolic treatment

B there is a fall in the plasma levels of cortisol, testosterone and aldosterone

C a woman is 2.5 kg heavier by 10 weeks compared with her non-pregnant weight

D at least 25% of all new mothers undergo a clinical postnatal depressive illness

E a frank puerperal psychosis is associated with a history of a traumatic termination of pregnancy, poor socioeconomic circumstances and perineal trauma

1.45 Puerperal sepsis

A endogenous infection is most likely from gastrointestinal flora
B a swinging pyrexia, hypotension and tachycardia are early signs
C prolonged bleeding in the postpartum period may indicate infection
D after a clinical diagnosis of puerperal infection, treatment should be deferred until antibiotic sensitivities are available
E an infected episiotomy may lead to a perineal abscess; this is treated by broad-spectrum antibiotics before sensitivities are known

1.46 The following are associated with premature labour

A obesity
B age under 15 years
C non-Caucasian
D presence of fibroids
E retained IUCD

1.47 The female breast

A alveoli are surrounded by oxytocin-sensitive contractile myoepithelial cells and each duct and ductule is lined by longitudinal contractile cells
B is influenced by a hormone manufactured by lactotrophs from the posterior pituitary, whose release is augmented by a neuroendocrine reflex
C during lactation releases 1400–1600 ml of milk per day
D milk letdown reflex is mediated by the decapeptide oxytocin
E shows significant hyperplasia and hypertrophy in pregnancy under the influence of oestrogen, growth hormone and dopamine

1.48 Thromboembolism and pregnancy

A risk increases with maternal age
B warfarin is teratogenic
C prolonged use of subcutaneous heparin is associated with vertebral osteopaenia
D heparin crosses the placenta
E lupus anticoagulant is associated with thrombotic disease

1.49   Premature rupture of the membranes

    A accounts for 30% of preterm deliveries
    B is defined as rupture of the fetal membranes before 37 completed weeks
    C is associated with coital activity
    D phospholipase A_2-generating bacteria have been implicated
    E amniotic fluid if seen has a pH of less than 7.1 and is checked for by nitrazine sticks

1.50   Abdominal pain in pregnancy

    A uterine body pain has sensory afferents from T6 to L2
    B due to pancreatitis there is a maternal mortality of 1%
    C due to renal calculi has an incidence of 1:1500 pregnancies
    D porphyria is a rare cause
    E the diagnosis of appendicitis may be difficult because the gravid uterus compresses the appendix against the pelvic side wall

1.51   The following anomalies are commonly associated with antiepileptic drugs

    A cleft lip
    B neural tube defects
    C facial dysmorphism
    D urethral valves
    E gastroschisis

1.52   Maternal serum alphafetoprotein

    A is an alpha-globulin
    B is synthesized only in the yolk sac
    C optimum time for detection in maternal serum is 16 weeks
    D is raised in closed neural tube defects
    E is lowered in trisomy 18

1.53 In the process of labour

A primary dysfunctional labour is defined as a labour in which the active phase progresses at a rate of less than 1 cm/h

B secondary arrest can be due to CPD, malposition or deflexion of the presenting part

C oxytocin increases the amplitude and frequency of contractions, but not the duration

D the name Caldeyro-Barcia and the city of Montevideo are linked in the term Montevideo units

E there is no validated evidence that the latent phase of labour should last less than 6 hours

1.54 Puerperal sepsis

A particularly virulent infection may occur with beta-haemolytic streptococci of endogenous origin

B offensive lochia may be an early sign and warrants aggressive antibiotic therapy

C antibiotic prophylaxis is warranted in high-risk situations such as prior to evacuation of a retained placenta

D increased blood flow to the pelvis in the postpartum period may predispose to septic thrombosis of pelvic veins

E swinging pyrexia is a sign which should lead to a search for a septic focus

1.55 Biophysical screening

A craniospinal defects account for over 50% of fetal abnormalities

B the 'lemon' sign describes the shape of the head in spina bifida

C choroid plexus cysts are common and not significant

D anencephaly is described as the absence of the fetal cranial vault

E closed spina bifida has a worse prognosis than open

1.56 In a woman who has had a previous Caesarean section

A judicious IOL does not increase the rate of true uterine rupture

B a subsequent trial of labour should be terminated by Caesarean section if, after 6 hours of active labour, delivery is not imminent

C with a breech presentation at term, Caesarean section is the preferred mode of delivery

D epidural anaesthesia in a subsequent trial of labour is unsafe for the mother

E the perinatal mortality rate in a subsequent pregnancy is higher than when the mother has not had a previous Caesarean section

1.57 HIV and pregnancy

A the fetus of an HIV-positive mother has a risk of transplacental infection of over 90%

B the detection of HIV antibodies in the neonate signifies infection with HIV

C pregnancy increases the risk of HIV-positive mothers developing AIDS

D the main risk to the fetus in pregnancy is related to a high incidence of transplacental opportunistic infection

E babies of HIV-positive mothers are commonly growth retarded

1.58 Amniocentesis

A the spontaneous abortion rate is less than 1%

B is used to measure acetylcholinesterase levels

C is routinely offered to women with a family history of Down's syndrome

D has increased risk of pulmonary hypoplasia

E is associated with amniotic band formation

1.59 In the haemoglobinopathies

A heterozygous sickle cell disease carriers have little disability and have a relative resistance to malaria

B homozygous beta-thalassaemia patients are healthy at birth since HbF is produced normally

C Tay-Sachs disease is rare among Caucasians but may have a carrier rate as high as 1:30 in Ashkenazi Jews

D homozygous sickle cell disease patients are prone to oxidant stress and sickling crises under general anaesthesia

E iron chelation therapy is often necessary after the regular blood transfusions received by homozygous beta-thalassaemia patients

1.60 Anticoagulant therapy in pregnancy

A warfarin therapy at 6–9 weeks gestation is associated with facial anomalies in the fetus

B oral warfarin may be commenced in the second trimester and continued until delivery

C long-term warfarin therapy is associated with an increased fetal mortality

D the anticoagulant effects of heparin are easily reversed with protamine sulphate

E oral heparin is recommended in the first trimester as it does not cross the placenta

PRACTICE PAPER TWO

Allow 1 hour for the completion of all 60 questions

Answers are on p. 105

2.1 Amniotic fluid embolus

A commonly associated with small uterine tears F
B the coagulation abnormality is associated with thromboplastic activity of amniotic fluid T
C fetal squames can be found in blood from the maternal right atrium T
D results in less than 60% mortality F
E immediate delivery is essential T

2.2 When a maternal death occurs

A the Enquiry Form MCW97 is sent to all health staff involved in the care of the woman, including midwives, general practitioners and obstetricians T
B the Regional Medical Officer of Health compiles the Report and forwards it to the Regional Obstetric Assessor
C the Regional Obstetric Assessor's Report may include reports from the Regional Anaesthetic Assessor, the District Coroner and the Regional Pathology Assessor
D a single main cause is allotted and classified according to the WHO International Classification of Diseases, 9th Revision, 1975 (ICD 9)
E all individuals involved in the care of the dead woman meet with the Assessors and discuss the Report

2.3 Preconceptual assessment

A a family history of congenital anomaly is an indication for genetic counselling T
B it is advisable for epileptics to change their medication to carbamazepine where possible T
C it is reasonable to intensify steroid therapy before pregnancy in patients with inflammatory bowel disease to achieve prolonged remission T
D optimal diabetic control in the preconceptual phase reduces the incidence of congenital anomalies T
E folic acid is recommended to all preconceptual women to reduce the risk of neural tube defects T

2.4 The following statements concern epidural anaesthesia

A sepsis is a contraindication T

B a platelet count above $80 \times 10^{12}/l$ is needed T(?)

3.

C incidence of dural tap can be up to 20% T

D postepidural headaches occur in up to 70% of cases F T

E Mendelson's syndrome is a rare complication T F

2.5 In assessing the human genome

A the PCR is a process to amplify specifically a short region of RNA for closer analysis F

B the identification of the F_{508} mutation in either parent may aid in the diagnosis of cystic fibrosis F (?) T

C the $\alpha°$-thalassaemia mutation can be identified by abnormal fragments on a Northern blot analysis F (?)

D Duchenne's muscular dystrophy is an ultimately lethal, X-linked disease affecting 1:3500 newborn female babies F

E there is an association between choroid plexus cysts, congenital heart disease and trisomy 18 T

4

2.6 The diagnosis of pregnancy

A increased pigmentation of the nipples occurs at 8 weeks and constitutes Montgomery's sign T F

B the nausea and vomiting of early pregnancy is confined to mornings F

C tingling of the breasts is an early sign T

D a commercially available pregnancy test may be positive before the first missed period, i.e. at 4 weeks gestation T

E the alpha subunit of hCG is specific and is measured by standard pregnancy tests F

4.

2.7 Placenta praevia

A incidence of approximately 0.4% T

B associated with increasing maternal age T

C more common in first pregnancies F (?)

5

D diagnosis is confirmed by ultrasound T

E can result in IUGR T

2.8 In the fetal circulation

A there is a primitive blood circulatory system developed by the end of the third embryonic week F T

B the right atrial crista dividens preferentially diverts blood from the superior vena cava through into the right ventricle F

C pulmonary artery blood flow is low because of the very high pulmonary artery vascular resistance T

D the blood is 80% saturated with oxygen as it leaves the placenta in the umbilical artery F (F)

E the ductus arteriosus preferentially diverts blood from the main pulmonary artery across to the aortic arch T

2.9 Analgesic therapy in pregnancy

A high-dose aspirin is recommended to reduce the severity of pre-eclampsia F

B non-steroidal agents cause premature closure of the fetal ductus arteriosus T

C obstetric haemorrhage may be potentiated by concomitant non-steroidal analgesic therapy T

D opiate-induced neonatal respiratory depression is readily reversible with naloxone T

E opiate therapy predisposes to gastric stasis and aspiration pneumonitis T

2.10 The following concern the biophysical profile

A fetal tone is an important component T

B chronic hypoxia will affect fetal breathing movements first F

C the biophysical profile is useful from 24 weeks onwards F T

D its use in high-risk pregnancies significantly reduces fetal demise T

E acute hypoxia is associated with loss of fetal heart rate accelerations T

2.11 An insulin-dependent diabetic in pregnancy

A has a 10% chance of having a fetus with a major congenital abnormality F

B with good blood glucose control, significantly decreases her risk of miscarriage in early pregnancy, especially if such control was achieved preconceptually T

C who delivers at 37 weeks may have a baby with significant RDS as hyperglycaemia inhibits surfactant production T

D does not need an ophthalmological opinion if she has had one within the past 3 years T

E is no more prone to develop pre-eclampsia than her non-diabetic counterpart F

2.12 Puerperal psychosis

A affects 1–2% of new mothers   T

B is commoner in those who continue to breast feed beyond 3 months   T

C may be precipitated by a trial of forceps   T

D should never be treated by electroconvulsive therapy   F

E is uncommon in more mature mothers   F

2.

2.13 The following are associated with breech presentation

A prematurity   T

B flexed legs   T

C anencephaly   T

D polyhydramnios   T

E cystic hygroma   T

4.

2.14 Fetomaternal haemorrhage and blood group incompatibility in pregnancy

A the Kleihauer test demonstrates the presence of fetal red blood cells in the maternal circulation   T

B an immunofluorescent test makes it possible to distinguish between maternally-derived HbF and fetally-derived HbF   ? f.

C ABO blood group incompatibility between the parents is the commonest cause of haemolytic disease of the newborn and erythroblastosis fetalis   T

D a normal vaginal delivery does not put a rhesus-negative mother at risk of isoimmunization   F

E maternally-derived IgM antibodies against fetal red blood cells may cross the placenta, leading to haemolysis of fetal red blood cells   F

4.

2.15 Caesarean section

A trial of scar is contraindicated if the section was via a classical incision   T

B the incidence of scar dehiscence in labour after a lower segment procedure is less that 0.5%   T (?)

C ureteric injury is more likely during a classical than a lower segment section   F

D the so-called 'crash' section should always be a classical Caesarean   F

E it is mandatory to 'lock' the first layer when suturing a lower segment incision   F

5

2.16   The following concern cephalopelvic disproportion

A women less than 155 cm tall have a greater risk of developing CPD T
B a high head at term is uncommon in Afro-Caribbean women F
C engagement of the head should occur before 39 weeks F   S
D diabetic patients are more prone to CPD T
E Bandl's ring can occur before uterine rupture T (?)

2.17   The onset of labour

A involves a cascade of chemicals in its primary initiation and, in particular, prostaglandin stimulation of the uterus secondary to uterine oxytocin priming F
B must be thought of as involving the mother and the fetus acting independently, rather than in concert F (?)
C probably occurs via prostaglandins stimulating the release of calcium ions from the uterine sarcoplasmic reticulum via a second messenger T
D will be preceded by a decrease in the amount of connective tissue in the cervix, leading to a massive decrease in cervical compliance and then cervical dilatation F
E shows a clear inverse relationship with the Bishop score of the cervix F T   (?)

2.18   Normal labour

A commences with the onset of regular painful contractions in the presence of a dilated cervix F progressive dilation
B retraction of the head during the second stage suggests an undiagnosed malposition T F
C the average time for the second stage is 1 hour in the multiparous woman F (?)
D nipple stimulation is an accepted part of physiological management of the third stage F ? T
E signs of placental separation include a gush of bright red placental blood X   F

2.19   Development of the female genital tract

A the genital ridge is the same in both sexes T
B the paramesonephric ducts will form the uterus, Fallopian tubes and cervix T
C the vagina develops from the urogenital sinus T
D the paramesonephric ducts are medial to the mesonephric ducts T
E the broad ligament develops from mesenchyme (?) T

2.20 Neonatal RDS

A may be beneficially treated with artificial surfactant T

B can be avoided or diminished in severity by administering antenatal
dexamethasone to the mother T

C has a frequency in term infants of 1% F

D complications include pulmonary interstitial emphysema, retinopathy of
prematurity and necrotizing pneumonitis T F

E may appear as a generalized reticulogranular opacity of the lungs on a
CXR, thereby resembling a 'snowstorm' T

4

2.21 Multiple pregnancy

A the incidence of twin pregnancy in the UK is 1 in 80 T   S

B perinatal mortality is increased in triplet pregnancy by a factor of ten T

C intrauterine growth retardation is common and is the main aetiological
factor in the increased perinatal mortality rate T F

D some obstetricians recommend prophylactic cervical cerclage in triplet
pregnancy T

E the outcome of triplet pregnancy is primarily related to fetal size at
delivery T F

2

2.22 The fetal hydantoin syndrome is associated with

A cleft lip and palate T

B hypospadias T

C club foot T

D growth retardation T

E nail and digital hypoplasia T

4

2.23 Cardiovascular changes in a normal singleton pregnancy

A include a generalized vasodilatation secondary to increased synthesis of the
vasodilatory prostaglandins E2 and prostacyclin F ? T

B result in a physiological haemodilutional anaemia with a lower limit of
10.5 g/dl T f 11g

C involve a 10% increase in stroke volume and a 15 bpm increase in pulse
rate T

D will result in a cardiac output of 9 l/min in the second stage T

E dictate a regular assessment of the diastolic blood pressure when the fifth
Korotkoff sound should be used F

2.24 Rhesus disease

A inheritance of the D antigen has a multifactorial mechanism

B complications of labour with a rhesus-affected fetus are those of macrosomia

C kernicterus in the neonate is a serious complication related to the degree of haemolysis

D estimation of bilirubin concentration from amniotic fluid is by change in optical density at 453 nm

E active immunization by anti-D is recommended for rhesus-negative mothers for any antenatal vaginal bleeding

2.25 In forceps delivery

A sciatic nerve injury can occur

B haematuria can result

C perineal damage is more common with the use of a ventouse

D fetal jaundice is common postdelivery

E cephalohaematomas commonly occur over the frontal bone

2.26 In a woman with eclampsia

A 50% of convulsions are postnatal, generally within 24 hours of delivery

B immediate delivery is vital to avoid any hypoxic cerebral damage to the mother and fetus

C magnesium carbonate is advocated by some authorities as the anticonvulsant of choice

D epidural analgesia may be safely used if the labour is induced, provided the platelet count is greater than $100 \times 10^{12}/l$

E there is always a prodromal phase, with symptoms of headache, epigastric pain and vomiting

2.27 Haemoglobinopathies

A sickle cell crises are less common in pregnancy

B heterozygous haemoglobin S and C (SC disease) patients have a mild form of sickle cell anaemia unaffected by pregnancy

C haemoglobin S and thalassaemia may coexist in the heterozygous state giving the clinical picture of sickle cell disease

D alpha-thalassaemia major leads to chronic anaemia and pregnancy is unlikely in these patients

E thalassaemia is a term given to anaemias with defective production of the haem moiety of haemoglobin

2.28 In the fetus

A there is a 40% risk of transplacental transmission of toxoplasmosis to the fetus if the mother has a primary infection in the pregnancy

B congenital toxoplasmosis is manifest by a classic triad of hydrocephalus, chorioretinitis and intracranial calcification

C with red blood cell alloimmunization, an intrauterine transfusion with group O, rhesus-negative blood compatible with maternal blood may be useful

D with posterior urethral valves, a vesicoamniotic shunt may be useful to decrease the associated lung hypoplasia

E infected with parvovirus, the evidence is that, if the fetus survives the initial viral infection, there are no long-term sequelae

2.29 In operative vaginal delivery

A station of the fetal head is defined as the distance in inches between the leading bony portion of the fetal skull and the plane of the maternal ischial spines

B when forceps are applied in the mid-pelvis, asynclitism and deflexion often require correction

C skull fracture, cephalohaematoma and subgaleal haemorrhage can occur in vacuum extraction

D mild neonatal jaundice and fetal scalp injuries are more common with forceps than the vacuum extractor

E the final position of the forceps on the fetal head must be biparietal and bimalar

2.30 Hypertonic uterine activity

A is the commonest form of abnormal uterine function in labour

B is more likely as a result of prostaglandin administration than with oxytocic agents

C hypertonic uterine activity as a result of placental abruption may be reversed with intravenous salbutamol

D in the absence of fetal distress, idiopathic hypertonicity as a result of oxytocin administration may be allowed to reverse spontaneously after stopping the infusion of the oxytocic

E is related to stress in the labouring woman

2.31 Intrauterine death

A coagulopathy can occur after 16 weeks if the fetus is retained for greater than 4 weeks
B fibrinogen falls at a rate of 50 mg/dl per week
C 90% of patients deliver within 1 week
D maternal blood group and antibodies should be taken
E maternal and paternal karyotypes should always be determined

2.32 To help in the diagnosis of hydrops fetalis

A symphysis fundal height is increased by at least 3 cm above expected
B liquor pool depth is between 4 and 6 cm
C oedema of the scalp is pathognomonic
D diaphragmatic hernia is always present
E cordocentesis is mandatory

2.33 Diagnostic events in early pregnancy occur at the following times

A increased nipple pigmentation at 8 weeks
B urinary frequency at the time of the missed period
C amenorrhoea 28 days postfertilization
D softening of the uterus and cervix at 6 weeks
E a beta-hCG level of 25–50 IU per litre at 10 days postfertilization

2.34 Intrauterine growth retardation

A can be defined as a birthweight below the 10th percentile for gestational age and sex
B is associated with significant neonatal morbidity
C results in hypoglycaemia and polycythaemia in the neonate
D is best detected by the use of symphysis–fundal height measurements
E is more common in lower socioeconomic groups

2.35 In pregnancy

A there is trophoblast invasion of the maternal placental bed as part of the paternal vascular response to placentation F

B the normal amniotic fluid depth at 36 weeks is between 2 and 10 cm F

C abnormal flow velocity waveforms in the uterine arteries recorded by Doppler USS are associated with proteinuric pregnancy-induced hypertension T

D risk factors for thromboembolic disease include positive lupus anticoagulant factor, obesity and immobilization T (4)

E amniotic fluid embolus is associated with excess uterine activity, late rupture of the membranes in labour and symptomatic oligohydramnios T (?) polyhydramnios

2.36 Episiotomy

A is recommended as an elective procedure where the mother is known to have berry aneurysms F T

B is commonly performed when premature babies deliver vaginally F T

C tearing of the anal musculature constitutes a third-degree tear F F

D incision of the posterior fourchette predisposes to excess scar tissue formation F

E interrupted chromic catgut sutures are recommended to minimise early discomfort F 2

2.37 Postpartum haemorrhage

A is more common following LSCS T

B occurs in 9% of pregnancies T

C can occur following nifedipine treatment T S.

D is associated with oligohydramnios F

E is more common in the presence of previous history of PPH T

2.38 In the female bony pelvis

A the anteroposterior inlet is represented by a straight line drawn from the lower anterior border of the sacral promontory to the anterior border of the symphysis pubis and is bordered laterally by the ileopectineal lines F

B the anteroposterior inlet and outlet should each be at least 11.0 cm if the pelvis is to be considered adequate for a vaginal delivery T 11 5cm

C a platypelloid shape has a short anteroposterior diameter, a narrow sacrosciatic notch with a predisposition to deep transverse arrest of the head F

D the pudendal nerve re-enters the pelvis via the lesser sciatic foramen lying lateral to the internal pudendal artery

E in the anatomical position the angle of inclination should be 150°

2.39 Infection in pregnancy

A maternal transmission of hepatitis B is more likely if the mother is
E antigen positive   T

B spread of hepatitis B is via infected blood and commonly occurs in the
neonatal period F

C the presence of antibody to hepatitis B in the 6-month-old infant signifies
infection F

D the HIV virus crosses the placenta   T

E the neonate may acquire HIV from breast milk T

2.40 In the management of premature labour

A corticosteroids are administered before 34 weeks   T

B chorioamnionitis is the only absolute contraindication to tocolysis F

C inhibition of labour beyond 34 weeks is contraindicated T

D ethanol can be used to suppress labour F   T

E all infants before 34 weeks gestation should be delivered by LSCS F

2.41 Maternal hyperthyroidism in pregnancy

A is associated with increased rates of cerebral palsy in the offspring F T

B when appropriately treated may cause spontaneous abortion and IUGR   T

C is best treated surgically as the drug of choice is teratogenic F

D is associated with hydatidiform mole due to very high levels of hCG F T

E may necessitate the use of propranolol and thyroxine during treatment T

2.42 Cancer in pregnancy

A the prognosis of breast cancer is unaltered by pregnancy F

B chemotherapy for Hodgkin's disease invariably renders the patient infertile F

C the natural history of malignant melanoma is adversely affected by
pregnancy F T

D the raised gonadotrophin levels in pregnancy have an adverse effect on
hormone-dependent thyroid cancer   T

E further pregnancy is contraindicated after successful treatment for breast
cancer F

2.43 Premature rupture of the membranes

A precedes 60% of singleton spontaneous preterm deliveries

B corticosteroid administration is contraindicated following PROM

C is associated with fetal pulmonary hypoplasia

D can result in an increased incidence of congenital dislocation of the hip

E has an increased risk of fetal distress

2.44 In non-immune hydrops fetalis

A it is believed that there are three main causes—anaemia, cardiac failure and hepatic failure

B maternal polyhydramnios and problems with the third stage are quite common

C chromosomal anomalies lie second only to the fetal cardiovascular system as a cause

D B and M mode echocardiography and fetal blood sampling are necessary to make the diagnosis

E transplacental drug treatments using digoxin, verapamil, amiodarone and flecainide have been advocated

2.45 Monitoring in labour

A continuous external cardiotocography is the preferred method of fetal monitoring in a high-risk labour in the presence of ruptured membranes

B intermittent auscultation gives comparable results to continuous external cardiotocography in terms of fetal outcome in low-risk labour

C a pH reading of 7.28 from a fetal blood sample in the latter period of the first stage of labour warrants urgent delivery

D complicated baseline bradycardia is the CTG pattern which correlates closest with a hypoxic fetal blood sample

E the pH value of fetal capillary blood falls by around 0.12 units/hour during the second stage of labour

2.46 The following cause a raised maternal serum AFP

A twins

B Turner's syndrome

C intrauterine death

D Down's syndrome

E non-Caucasian women

2.47 In pregnancy

A prescribing chloramphenicol for the mother in the second trimester is safer for the fetus, than if given to the mother in the third trimester

B maternal intrapartum penicillin prophylaxis effectively prevents vertical transmission of Group B streptococci

C Caesarean section less than 4 hours from rupture of the membranes is the preferred mode of delivery in cases of primary active genital herpes

D a mother who develops acute toxoplasmosis in which the fetus is affected should be treated with spiramycin, pyrimethamine and sulphonamides

E there are good arguments in favour of giving prophylactic antibiotics to all women undergoing Caesarean section

2.48 Preconceptual assessment

A the input of a clinical geneticist is recommended

B preconceptual counselling after a traumatic delivery is likely to have a negative effect

C the diabetic patient should be advised to book early in pregnancy with a view to stabilizing blood sugar levels within a narrow range

D it is mandatory to alter drug prescriptions where there is a risk of congenital malformation

E stable cardiac disease with no adverse symptoms will not be adversely affected by pregnancy

2.49 Concerning biophysical screening

A cystic hygroma is always associated with Turner's syndrome

B duodenal atresia is associated with trisomy 21 in 30% of cases

C diaphragmatic hernia is non-recurrent

D gastroschisis is associated with chromosomal anomalies in 30% of cases

E omphalocele is a midline defect covered in peritoneum

2.50 In pregnancy

A the fetus is at risk of injury in a road traffic accident in three ways—direct trauma, indirect trauma and deceleration injury

B the most common cause of non-obstetric trauma is road traffic accidents

C there is an 80% fetal loss rate after a road traffic accident from which the mother develops hypovolaemic shock

D a combination diagonal shoulder to waist and lap seat belt should be worn with the straps above and below 'the bump' of the pregnancy

E after a road traffic accident fetomaternal haemorrhage is more common with an anteriorly located placenta

2.51 Anaemia related to pregnancy

A is defined as a haemoglobin level less that 11.0 g/dl

B if a patient is iron deficient in the second trimester then fetal uptake of her iron stores is likely to be the main cause

C women with oligomenorrhoea are more likely to become iron deficient in pregnancy

D eating red meat is an efficient method of obtaining dietary iron

E a reduction in serum ferritin below the normal range is a late manifestation of iron-deficiency anaemia and suggests refractory anaemia

2.52 Chorionic villus sampling

A can only be performed transabdominally

B has a spontaneous abortion rate of approximately 4%

C is associated with limb and facial deformities if performed before 10 weeks

D results are available within 24 hours

E is most useful in patients with high recurrence rate

2.53 In malpresentations and malpositions of the fetus

A breech extraction is a safe option in a singleton pregnancy

B where there is an upper limb beside the fetal head, Caesarean section is necessary

C with a face presentation, a vaginal delivery is possible, provided it is mentoposterior

D where there is a brow presenting, rotational forceps are an option for delivery

E there is an association with a gynaecoid pelvis

2.54 Disseminated intravascular coagulation in pregnancy

A occasionally has a primary haematological cause

B effects are due to consumption of clotting factors and platelets

C the risk of DIC increases with time if a dead fetus is not delivered

D adequate replacement therapy includes injection of calcium ions

E intravenous heparin has a place in management when there is an intact circulation

2.55 Placental abruption

A occurs in 1% of pregnancies T
B is associated with a decreased AFP F
C can result in a Couvelaire uterus T
D is associated with premature labour T
E is more common in oligohydramnios F

2.56 Amniocentesis

A should only be performed after informed consent is obtained T
B has a fetal loss rate of 1% T
C can safely be performed as a 'blind' procedure F
D may be indicated if there is a family history of Duchenne's muscular
     dystrophy T
E and bilirubin levels are associated with Liley curves T

2.57 Adverse drug reactions in pregnancy include

A tetracyclines and staining of fetal teeth T
B ibuprofen and premature closure of the ductus arteriosus T
C pethidine and maternal gastric stasis T
D naloxone and inhibition of fetal respiration F
E aspirin and postpartum haemorrhage T

2.58 Oligohydramnios

A defined as liquor with a pool depth less than 2 cm T
B associated with a decreased AFP F
C results in an increased perinatal mortality by 40-fold ? T
D requires regular fetal assessment T
E is more common in multiple pregnancy F

2.59 In a pregnant epileptic

A the risk of the fetus being born with epilepsy is 1:80 T 1:40.
B phenytoin is the drug of choice F
C there is an association with vitamin B12 deficiency F
D anticonvulsant levels can be monitored from maternal saliva samples F T
E there is a three-fold increase in the rate of abruption T

2.60 Thalassaemia

A the alpha-globin chains are specified by four genes, two from each parent T

B alpha-thalassaemia major occurs when no alpha chains are formed ? T

C severe pre-eclampsia is associated with a fetus having no alpha chain-producing genes F T

D after antenatal diagnosis of a fetus with beta-thalassaemia major, parents are informed that it is incompatible with life F

E a patient with beta-thalassaemia minor may present for the first time in pregnancy T

PRACTICE PAPER THREE

Allow 1 hour for the completion of all 60 questions

Answers are on p. 111

3.1 The following are associated with amniotic fluid embolus

A uterine stimulation   T
B large babies   T
C intrauterine death   F
D right ventricular strain on ECG   T
E perihilar infiltrates on CXR   T

4

3.2 During and after delivery of the fetus

A lung aeration causes a marked decrease in pulmonary vascular resistance   F   T
   with concomitant increases in pulmonary blood flow and left atrial pressure
B thoracic compression and a drop in temperature, pCO_2 and pH lead to initiation of respiration   F
C the umbilical arteries will eventually form the lateral umbilical ligaments   *medial*
   and superior vesical arteries   D   F
D placental occlusion will cause a rise in IVC blood pressure   F   f   2
E assessment of the neonate born with meconium liquor necessitates a paediatric opinion   T ✓

3.3 Malpresentation of the fetus

A is associated with an increased risk of congenital anomaly   T
B compound presentation precludes a vaginal delivery   F
C commonly occurs in association with an anthropoid pelvis   F   F *malposition.*
D may be corrected during labour by intravenous oxytocic agents   F
E should be treated by immediate stabilizing induction if the membranes rupture   f

4

3.4 Anaesthesia in pregnancy

A cricoid pressure is essential before induction of general anaesthesia

B aortocaval compression is minimized by right lateral tilt

C Mendelson's syndrome is a risk during general anaesthetic

D previous Caesarean section is a contraindication to an epidural

E epidural anaesthesia results in a higher forceps rate

3.5 A pregnant diabetic woman

A should be delivered by 39 weeks because of the risk of stillbirth if she continues beyond this

B in labour needs continuous maternal and fetal monitoring

C in labour should ideally have a blood glucose of 6–8 mmol/l with a sliding scale insulin regimen charted

D has a fetus at increased risk of developing jaundice because polycythaemia and hyperbilirubinaemia are more common in such fetuses

E has a fetus with a 10-fold increased risk of developing diabetes in later life

3.6 Antibiotic prophylaxis against puerperal sepsis should be considered

A after forceps delivery in a diabetic patient

B in a patient with a history of pelvic sepsis

C after ventouse delivery

D after four vaginal examinations in the first stage of labour with intact membranes

E after episiotomy in a patient with chronic anaemia

3.7 The following concern antepartum haemorrhage

A vasa praevia is a rare cause

B fetal blood cells can be detected by sodium hydroxide

C PPH is a well-known association

D abruption results in painless vaginal bleeding

E occurs at some time in 20% of pregnancies

3.8 Induction of labour

A may be defined as an obstetric procedure designed to preempt the natural process of labour by initiating its onset artificially before this occurs spontaneously T

B will involve an increase in the concentration of bound calcium ions in the sarcoplasmic reticulum of the uterine smooth muscle F

C with prostaglandins has a 0.1% risk of uterine hypertonus F

D will result in a decreased incidence of neonatal hyponatraemia when prostaglandins alone are used T

E carries a theoretical risk of premature closure of the ductus arteriosus if prostaglandins are used F

3.9 Uterine activity in labour

A the commonly accepted unit of measurement is kPa/30 min F

B the myometrium acts as a syncytium T

C idiopathic uterine hypotonicity in a primigravid patient is generally easily overcome by intravenous oxytocic agents T

D hypotonicity may be postural T

E uterine pressure waves are generated from the fundus T

usually

5

3.10 Biophysical profile

A is made up of four components F

B a score of 6 or more is always satisfactory T F *cot of olygohydamnios*

C perinatal mortality rises with falling biophysical profile score T

D amniotic fluid volume is an important sign of acute asphyxia F

E consists of Doppler flow readings of the umbilical cord F

4

3.11 In a woman with a normal singleton pregnancy

A the transverse diameter of the thorax increases with an elevation and increased excursion of the diaphragm F *constant.*

B the respiratory tidal volume, the respiratory rate and vital capacity all increase, resulting in a hyperventilatory state F

C there is a mild alkalaemia with an arterial pH of 7.44 T

D gastric secretion and motility are decreased and salivary excretion is increased T

E the raised alkaline phosphatase is mostly placental in origin T

5

3.12 Malposition of the fetus

A may be diagnosed antenatally and is an indication for induction F

B occipitoposterior position is an absolute indication for augmentation of labour F

C a baby in the occipitoposterior position may be delivered by non-rotational forceps T

D a face presentation may result in spontaneous vaginal delivery T.

E most brow presentations are delivered by Caesarean section T

S

3.13 Management of a breech presentation

A extension of the fetal head is a contraindication for vaginal delivery T.

B estimation of fetal weight by USS is mandatory T   ? F

C augmentation with Syntocinon is contraindicated in a breech F.

D inlet and outlet should both be greater than 11.5 cm in diameter T

E a flat sacrum is the ideal pelvic shape F

3.14 In the hypertensive disorders of pregnancy

4

A phaeochromocytoma is best treated with an alpha-adrenergic blockade before delivery T

B the HELLP syndrome (haematemesis, elevated liver enzymes and low platelets) may complicate the picture F

C the recurrence rate of pre-eclampsia after one affected pregnancy is of the order of 5% T   75 m/r

D low-dose aspirin, (150 mg/day, may be of benefit T   F

E pre-eclampsia is definitely due to altered uterine spiral artery function F

4.

3.15 Infection of the fetus during pregnancy

A deafness is the most likely consequence of rubella infection in late pregnancy T

B once maternal immunity to cytomegalovirus is acquired there is no risk to the fetus F.

C toxoplasmosis may be suspected if the mother has a non-specific illness with generalized lymphadenopathy T

D congenital infection with toxoplasmosis is associated with fetal anomaly in the majority of cases F

E varicella zoster crosses the placenta T

4

3.16 Cephalopelvic disproportion in a primigravid patient can be suspected in the following situations

A cervical dilatation stops at 7 cm
B the cervix is well applied to the presenting part
C recurrent deep decelerations on the CTG occur
D prolonged pregnancy
E prolonged latent phase

3.17 Investigations in the hypertensive disorders of pregnancy

A can involve research-based angiotensin infusion pressor studies in the pregnant mother
B to assess hepatic function include aspartate aminotransferase, total protein, urate, creatinine and albumin
C which reveal a significant urinary vanillyl mandelic acid level warrant immediate consultant-led management
D should always include assessments of fetal wellbeing and growth
E may show a microcytic thrombocytopenia

3.18 The rhesus-negative mother

A is very likely to possess the δ antigen on chromosome 1
B should be offered chorionic villus sampling if previously sensitized to the rhesus factor
C should have antibody titres measured by direct Coomb's test with dilutional titres if detected
D has a 50% chance of sensitization to the D antigen if exposed to fetal blood where the father is homozygous D positive
E if antibody negative at booking will require repeat antenatal antibody estimation only if there is antepartum haemorrhage

3.19 Development of the urinary system

A the epoophoron is a remnant of the mesonephros
B the paroophoron lies medial to the ovary
C the urinary system arises from the intermediate cell mass
D the urethra develops in part from the metanephros
E the allantois degenerates to form the urachus

3.20 The pharmaceutical treatment of hypertension in pregnancy

A should always be commenced after two BP readings of
   greater than 140/90 mmHg
B with IV hydralazine should control the BP within 5 minutes
C rarely may involve sodium nitroprusside
D with nifedipine may initially induce significant headache due to its
   vasodilatory mode of action
E should normally be continued for at least 2–3 weeks after discharge from
   hospital before it is decreased or stopped

3.21 Infection and pregnancy

A a febrile illness may precipitate premature labour
B vaginal beta-haemolytic streptococci have a prevalence of 9% in pregnancy
C pregnant women with a history of genital herpes should have regular vaginal swabs in late pregnancy
D in the presence of active genital herpes, Caesarean section is the preferred
   mode of delivery where the membranes have been ruptured for over 4
   hours
E neonatal herpes is an unlikely outcome of vaginal delivery in the presence
   of active herpes provided it is a primary attack

3.22 The following concern epileptic mothers

A folate deficiency is associated with anticonvulsant therapy
B maternal epilepsy is associated with an increase in early pregnancy bleed-
   ing
C CTGs are unaffected by anticonvulsants
D they have a three-fold increase in breech presentation
E cardiovascular malformations are increased four-fold

3.23 In an obstructed labour

A the classic evidence for CPD is progressive moulding and caput during
   labour accompanied by true descent of the presenting part
B a persistent occipitotransverse position in a platypelloid pelvis indicates a
   trial of Kielland's forceps
C the critical denominator is the position of the true midpoint of the fetal
   head, the BPD
D a true contracted pelvis with an average-size fetus is a rare cause of CPD
E the use of oxytocin and epidural anaesthesia are associated with an
   increased incidence of instrumental delivery

3.24 Cancer in pregnancy

A stage I cancer of the cervix in the third trimester is managed by Caesarean delivery, then interval radical hysterectomy at 6 weeks *T* *F*

B the prognosis for cervical cancer is worse in pregnancy *F*

C there are over 400 reported cases of vulval cancer in pregnancy *T* *F*

D a reasonable interval of 2 years after treatment of Hodgkin's disease is recommended before a patient attempts to conceive *F* *T*

E radiotherapy for Hodgkin's lymphoma of the hilar nodes is an indication for termination of the pregnancy *F*

3.

3.25 In operative vaginal deliveries

A ventouse is associated with an increased requirement of anaesthesia *T*

B forceps delivery results in a three-fold increase in perineal trauma when compared with a ventouse *T*

C forceps result in a higher perinatal morbidity *T*

D a chignon lasts for approximately 48 hours *T*

E skull fractures will be linear rather than depressed *T* *5*

3.26 The renal system in pregnancy (16)

A the GFR is 60% greater than normal by 12 weeks *F*

B there is a link between UTI and low birthweight and preterm labour *T*

C acute glomerulonephritis is a rare condition and is usually initially diagnosed as pre-eclampsia *T*

D asymptomatic bacteriuria has a frequency of 5% and a prevalence of 1.2% *F* *T*

E the creatinine and urea decrease in the normal woman compared with non-pregnant values *T* *4*

3.27 Monitoring in labour (high)

A cardiotocography has a low false-positive rate *F* *F* *F* ✓

B monitoring of the growth-retarded fetus is by intermittent auscultation *F*

C cardiotocography plus fetal blood sampling is an ideal method of monitoring *F* ✓

D in low-risk labour it is acceptable to take CTG readings at 4-hourly intervals *T* ✓

E a fetal scalp electrode should be applied where possible in high-risk labour as it gives a more accurate CTG recording *F* *T* ✓ *5*

3.28 Hydrops fetalis is associated with

A pre-eclampsia
B fetal cardiac arrhythmias
C listeriosis
D trisomy 18
E rubella infection

3.29 Prenatal diagnosis

A maternal serum AFP results are expressed in multiples of the mean for unaffected pregnancies at that gestation
B a mother who has spina bifida has a 3–4% risk of having a fetus with a neural tube defect
C chorionic villus biopsy is associated with an excess risk of miscarriage, termination for abnormality and late fetal loss
D chorionic villus biopsy performed after 10 weeks gestation may result in the oromandibular limb hypoplasia syndrome
E as cystic fibrosis is an autosomal recessive condition, and 1 in 22 people in the UK are asymptomatic carriers, assuming no consanguinity, the chance of two such carriers mating is 1:484

3.30 Rhesus disease

A at least three genes, C, D and E, produce the rhesus antigen
B over 95% of cases of rhesus incompatibility relate to antibodies directed against the D antigen
C fetal haemolysis leads to appearances of growth retardation on ultrasonography
D fetal haemoglobin may be measured by cordocentesis and results plotted on to Liley charts
E undiagnosed rhesus disease may present with evidence of fetal distress on CTG

3.31 In the management of intrauterine death

A prostaglandin administration is associated with a rise in temperature
B vaginal delivery is mandatory
C amniotomy is contraindicated
D hypertonic glucose solutions are contraindicated because of infection risk
E extra-amniotic infusions can be associated with abruption

3.32 In preterm labour and delivery

A women with two or more previous preterm births have an 80% chance of repeating the process

B the three most frequent associations are placentitis, funicitis and amnionitis

C approximately one-third are associated with preterm rupture of the membranes

D maternal colonization with *Ureaplasma urealyticus* is not significant

E rupture of the membranes is a prerequisite for intra-amniotic infection as bacteria are incapable of crossing intact membranes

3.33 Multiple pregnancy

A the incidence of triplet pregnancy in the UK would be 1 in 6400 if Hellin's law was obeyed

B the glomerular filtration rate is reduced

C locked twins are a common cause of perinatal mortality

D mothers with triplet pregnancy are usually admitted for bed rest in the third trimester due to the high incidence of hypertension

E malpresentation of the second twin is an indication for elective Caesarean section

3.34 The use of USS in the management of intrauterine growth retardation

A pregnancy can be diagnosed at 5 weeks

B the use of crown–rump measurements is accurate to within 7 days

C the biparietal measurement gives the best estimate of fetal weight

D symmetrical IUGR is associated with an extrinsic cause

E over 70% of IUGR fetuses are normal

3.35 In prenatal diagnosis

A a raised AFP may be due to an anterior abdominal wall defect

B an AFP of less than 0.4 MoMs is suggestive of Down's syndrome

C the normal diameter of the anterior horn of the lateral ventricles is less than 8 mm

D there is a single laterally placed cerebral ventricle in holoprosencephaly

E omphalocele has a better prognosis than gastroschisis

3.36 The diagnosis of pregnancy

A may be delayed as there is commonly a small blood loss at the time of the first missed period T

B nausea and vomiting usually precedes amenorrhoea F

C a portable Doppler ultrasound machine may detect a fetal heart at 6 weeks F

D in the absence of biophysical and biochemical diagnostic aids a bimanual examination to detect Hegar's sign should be performed F

E the beta subunit of hCG is similar to corresponding units on LH, FSH and TSH, giving false-positive results on immunosorbent assays F

5

3.37 Massive obstetric haemorrhage

A occurs with 15% or greater blood volume loss T

B can be treated with intramyometrial prostaglandins T

C uterine atony may require hysterectomy T

D internal iliac ligation is contraindicated F

E treatment should be multidisciplinary T

5

3.38 Chorionic villus biopsy

A is safer than amniocentesis F

B is associated with a spontaneous abortion rate of 1% T

C is performed at 8–11 weeks gestation F at 10/52

D may result in chimaerism in the tissue culture ? T

E can be safely performed transcervically F

3

mosacusm

3.39 Puerperal psychosis

A the commonest complaint is of feelings of rejection toward the baby T F

B identification of at-risk women should lead to their receiving the necessary support in the antenatal period and reduce the incidence of puerperal psychosis T

C lack of support from a partner is a common symptom F

D patients may present to a marriage guidance counsellor T

E antidepressant drugs should not be prescribed until the diagnosis is established after repeated consultations F

3

3.40 **Secondary postpartum haemorrhage**

A occurs after more than 5% of deliveries F
B results from infection of retained products T
C is rarely due to choriocarcinoma T
D usually occurs in the first week after delivery F   ? ? 2nd
E must be treated with broad-spectrum antibiotics before evacuation T

S.

3.41 **Postpartum haemorrhage**

A is mostly due to uterine atony T
B can be due to the vasodilator nifedipine T
C should always be treated by a blood transfusion if the loss is massive T F
D may lead to hysterectomy and external iliac artery ligation F
E has a 5% incidence 10 weeks postnatally F

4.

3.42 **Regarding coagulation and pregnancy**

A there is inhibition of fibrinolytic activity T
B there is loss of elastic and muscle tissue in uterine vessel walls to enhance
  blood flow T F
C at-risk patients should be admitted for bed rest F
D treatment of a suspected pulmonary embolus should be deferred until a
  ventilation–perfusion scan is obtained F
E a patient on warfarin in established labour should be promptly treated with
  protamine sulphate F

4.

3.43 **Premature labour**

A can result from infections with group B streptococcus T
B ß-adrenergic agonists can result in fetal hypoglycaemia F T
C cervical change must be present for the correct diagnosis T
D has a prevalence of up to 9% T
E is defined as regular uterine contractions productive of cervical change
  prior to 40 completed weeks of gestation F

S

3.44 In operative vaginal delivery

A Wrigley's forceps have a variable pivot lock and short handles and are out-let forceps F

B the classic method of application of Kielland's forceps is now considered unsafe ? T

C the vacuum extractor may be used for delivery before full dilatation T

D abdominal palpation revealing one-fifth palpable necessitates a Caesarean section F

E the seventh cranial nerve is at risk during a forceps delivery T

S

3.45 Cancer in pregnancy

A should be managed by the obstetrician in a district hospital F

B radical surgery for vulval cancer may be performed in the first half of preg-nancy and the pregnancy allowed to continue T

C pregnancy may continue during cytotoxic therapy provided that methotrex-ate is not part of the treatment regimen F

D TSH-dependent thyroid cancers are adversely affected by pregnancy T

E melanoma is the cancer most likely to metastasise to the placenta T

S

3.46 Premature rupture of the membranes

A regular monitoring of the patient's temperature is the best indication of infection T

B LSCS is indicated for all premature breech deliveries F

C results in an increased risk of cord prolapse T

D positional foot deformaties can result T

E uterine contractions are always present with PROM F

S

3.47 The diagnosis of pregnancy

A may be made by the presence of Montgomery's tubercles T F

B may be made before a missed period by specific ELISA methods detecting the alpha subunit of hCG F

C should always be confirmed by examining for Hegar's sign F

D by USS can be made at 5 weeks T

E by urinalysis may be missed due to bacteriuria F T

3

3.48 Rhesus haemolytic disease

A the affected fetus may be treated by intraperitoneal transfusion T

B amniocentesis is preferred to cordocentesis as a means of monitoring the degree of fetal haemolysis due to its greater accuracy F

C blood for intrauterine transfusion is screened for cytomegalovirus T

D if the diagnosis is made on biophysical investigation, the disease process is relatively advanced F T

E intrauterine transfusion is recommended if fetal haematocrit is less than 30% between 26 and 30 weeks gestation ? T

3.49 Biophysical screening

A posterior urethral valves occur exclusively in males F

B cardiac anomalies occur in approximately 8:1000 live births T

C omphalocele is associated with chromosomal anomalies in 30% of cases T

D oligohydramnios only occurs in renal agenesis F

E polyhydramnios is associated with any bowel obstruction F

3.50 Episiotomy

A is most commonly cut as a mediolateral incision F T

B is linked with dyspareunia and faecal incontinence T

C is best repaired using a continuous subcuticular suture T

D may involve fibres of bulbospongiosus and the sphincter vaginae T

E may be comfortably repaired under a pudendal nerve blockade T

3.51 Drug treatment in pregnancy

A erythromycin may be given for urinary infections in the penicillin-sensitive patient F T

B methotrexate may be given for a severe exacerbation of psoriasis F

C papaveretum (Omnopon) may be preferred to pethidine in early labour as it has a longer duration of action F

D sodium valproate is the antiepileptic agent of choice F

E low-dose aspirin may reduce the severity of pre-eclampsia due to its antiplatelet action T

3.52 Cordocentesis

A involves inserting a needle into the cord at its junction with the placenta $\top$
B is indicated for chromosomal assessment after failed amniocentesis $\top$
C is the first choice in management of metabolic disorders $\times$ F
D has 2% risk of fetal loss $\top$
E is used for transfusion in rhesus disease $\top$

4

3.53 When a woman is induced into labour

95%

A the use of prostaglandins followed by amniotomy and/or Syntocinon results in 85% of them going into established labour $\times$ F
B the use of vaginal prostaglandins is contraindicated in the presence of ruptured membranes F
C the umbilical cord gases of babies born to mothers who have undergone an induction of labour followed by a normal vaginal delivery, show significant differences to those whose mothers laboured and delivered spontaneously $\top$
D there is a 10% failure to establish labour F (2 — 5%)
E using prostaglandins administered by any route, it is known that prostaglandins wil cross the placenta into the fetal circulation $\top$

3

3.54 Uterine function in labour

A intrauterine pressure of 700 kPa/15 min is at the lower end of the normal range at the 10th centile F $\top$
B hypotonic uterine activity predisposes to fetal hypoxia by inhibiting uterine blood flow F
C it takes 30 minutes for the effect of oxytocic hyperstimulation to wear off after the infusion is stopped F
D hypertonic uterine activity is commonly idiopathic F F
E calculation of intrauterine pressure is independent of baseline uterine muscle tone F

3

3.55 Biochemical screening

A a low AFP level alone will detect 30% of Down's syndrome pregnancies $\top$
B a low hCG is associated with Down's syndrome F
C the triple test will detect over 70% of cases of Down's syndrome F
D a low oestriol is associated with Down's syndrome $\top$
E a high AFP is associated with bleeding in the first trimester $\top$

5

3.56 In preterm rupture of the membranes

A testing the pH of the liquor reveals a pH of 6.5 F
B examination of the liquor on a glass slide will show ferning F
C *E. coli*, coital activity and vaginal examination are implicated T
D regular monitoring of the maternal temperature is more diagnostic of infection than C-reactive protein and the ESR T
E oligohydramnios and congenital dislocation of the hip are associated T
S

3.57 Anaemia in pregnancy

A vitamin B12 stores are commonly exhausted in the pregnant state F
B folate deficiency is commoner in women of higher social class F
C folate therapy is particularly important in epileptic patients T
D commonly prescribed iron therapy in pregnancy also contains folate T
E megaloblastic anaemia is associated with neural tube defects T

3.58 Oligohydramnios is associated with

A pre-eclampsia T
B diabetes mellitus F
C postmaturity T
D trisomy 21 F
E intrauterine growth retardation T
4

3.59 Breech presentation

A vaginal examination is imperative at the time of membrane rupture to exclude cord prolapse T
B electronic fetal monitoring is advisable T
C epidural anaesthesia is contraindicated in breech presentation F
D Elkins' manoeuvre encourages spontaneous version T
E Syntocinon is indicated for delay in second stage F 1st stage only
3

3.60 Premature labour

A is more common in multigravidae F
B is associated with smoking T
C is preceded by ruptured membranes in over a third of cases T
D the use of MgSO$_4$ is contraindicated in myasthenia gravis T
E prostaglandin synthetase inhibitors can cause polyhydramnios F
4

PRACTICE PAPER FOUR

Allow 1 hour for the completion of all 60 questions

Answers are on p. 119

4.1 Vaginal hysterectomy

A is the most common operation performed for menorrhagia

B has a much lower morbidity rate than abdominal hysterectomy

C urinary retention is common postoperatively

D vault prolapse occurs following 20% of vaginal hysterectomies

E it is the treatment of choice for procidentia

4.2 In urogynaecology

A an unstable bladder is defined as one shown objectively to contract spontaneously or on provocation during the filling phase whilst the patient is
attempting to inhibit micturition

B the loss of social awareness of the need to be continent of urine is usually
associated with dementia or a space-occupying lesion of the frontal cortex

C urinary incontinence is defined as an involuntary loss of urine which is
subjectively demonstrable and a social or hygienic problem

D in the Western world urinary fistulae are usually iatrogenic

E approximately 25% of patients with urinary incontinence delay for 5 years
or more before seeking advice

4.3 Amenorrhoea

A when patients present in their mid-teens, a physiological delay is the most
likely explanation

B obstruction to menstrual flow is associated with virilization

C the patient should be informed of the diagnosis in all circumstances

D when there is absence of the lower genital tract the use of graduated vaginal dilators may give good results in the unmotivated patient

E there is a significant risk of malignant change in maldeveloped gonads

4.4 Spontaneous abortion

A is associated with chromosomal abnormalities in 50% of cases T

B is defined as the loss of a fetus or embryo weighing 500 g or less F/T *with definition*

C the incidence is approximately 60% F

D is threatened if the pregnancy is non-viable F

E the risk of abortion occurring after an ultrasound showing a viable fetus is less than 1% F ?

4

4.5 In detrusor instability

A the majority of women have a clearly delineated cause F

B the incidence decreases after incontinence surgery F

C coital incontinence is not found F

D imipramine is used particularly in the treatment of nocturia and nocturnal enuresis T

E it may occur in 10% of the population and be asymptomatic T

5

4.6 Sexually transmitted diseases

A as a result of modern screening policies congenital syphilis has been eradicated in the UK F

B pus from a Bartholin's abscess should be sampled with charcoal swabs and transported in Stuart's medium F T

C *Chlamydia trachomatis* consists of DNA and is an intracellular parasite F

D Chlamydial infection often coexists with syphilis F

E beta-lactamase positive strains of *Neisseria gonorrhoea* usually respond to treatment with penicillin F

4

4.7 Bartholin's glands

A are situated at the posterior parts of the labia majora T

B can get infected and result in abscess formation T

C excision of the cyst when infected is desirable F

D are commonly infected by staphylococci and gonococci T

E infected glands always require surgical drainage T f

4

4.8   In the soft tissues of the pelvis

A the urethra and internal anal sphincter are supplied by the pudendal nerve

B the urethra emerges at its external meatus between the origins of pubococcygeus

C the deep inguinal (femoral) lymph nodes are medial to the femoral vein

D adjacent to the bladder neck there is a true internal urethral sphincter giving urinary continence

E the ureter is most at risk of injury during oophorectomy as it crosses the
bifurcation of the internal iliac artery into its anterior and posterior divi-
sions

4.9   Vulval dystrophy

A human papilloma virus infection is an aetiological factor

B lichen sclerosus is commonly diagnosed by characteristic changes seen on
examination

C hypertrophic dystrophy is associated with flattening of rete ridges

D the presence of severe associated inflammation is an indication for the use
of testosterone cream

E skinning vulvectomy is used in severe cases with a high cure rate

4.10   The following may be associated with dyspareunia

A spasm of the pubococcygeus muscle

B Behçet's syndrome

C irritable bowel syndrome

D urethral caruncle

E pelvic inflammatory disease

4.11   The ureters

A are each about 35–40 cm long in the normal adult female

B cross in front of the genitofemoral nerves and are themselves crossed by
the ovarian vessels in their pelvic course

C have four layers: an outer fibrous, a muscularis, then an intima and finally
a mucosal layer

D are supplied by branches of the abdominal aorta, renal gonadal, common
iliac, internal iliac vesical and uterine arteries

E are innervated by the T11–L2 spinal cord segments

4.12 Male subfertility

A is a significant factor in 1 in 10 infertile couples F ✓
B psychosexual problems are a common male factor in infertility clinics ✗
C the presence of antisperm antibodies is commonly tested by a mixed agglu-
tinin reaction on a fresh semen sample T
D oligozoospermia of 10–20 million per ml may respond to measures such as
stopping smoking and reducing alcohol intake T
E certain infective agents may cause obstruction of the vas deferens, this is
diagnosed by vasography during surgical exploration T

4.

4.13 Factors predisposing to ectopic pregnancies include

A pelvic inflammatory disease especially with chlamydia and gonorrhoea T
B IUCD F.
C GIFT T
D combined oral contraceptive F.
E previous ectopic pregnancy T

5 ✓

4.14 In the adrenal glands

A androgens are secreted from the outer zona glomerulosa region ✗
B 50% of circulating testosterone in the female is derived from the adrenals, T
with 25% coming from the ovaries and 25% from extraglandular sources
C the blood supply comes from the abdominal aorta, the inferior phrenic
arteries and the renal arteries T
D the main androgen secreted during fetal life is dehydroepiandrosterone sulphate (DHEAS) T
E postmenopausal androgens are a more important source of oestrogen than
ovarian oestrogens T

3

4.15 Regarding endometriosis

A the most widely accepted theory is of embolization of endometrial cells F
B ectopic endometrium is not identical morphologically to eutopic
endometrium F. T
C high local concentrations of macrophages have been implicated in possible
mechanisms for the pain and infertility of endometriosis T
D retrograde menstruation in an immunologically susceptible woman can
cause endometriotic deposits T
E increased concentrations of prostaglandins in association with endometriosis inhibit ovum release and tubal motility T F

3

4.16 Fibroids

A occur in over 30% of women of reproductive age   T
B can undergo sarcomatous change in 2% of cases   F   0.2%.
C are always associated with menorrhagia   f.
D can cause polycythaemia   T
E can be attached to the bladder   T

4.17 Hirsutism

A is commonest in the third and fourth decades of life   T
B in Cushing's syndrome is associated with plethoric facies due to androgen-induced erythrocytosis   F   T   (?)
C a formal dexamethasone suppression test will help to distinguish between an adrenal tumour and adrenal hyperplasia   T
D the use of the antioestrogenic progestogen, cyproterone acetate, will often help the hirsutes to regress   F
E the potassium-sparing diuretic, spironolactone, can interfere with the sexual differentiation of a female fetus, if the patient becomes pregnant whilst taking the drug   F   T   *male fetus*   3.

4.18 Carcinoma of the ovary

A is predisposed to by prolonged use of the oral contraceptive pill   F
B cancers of epithelial origin comprise 90% of total primary malignancies   T
C borderline tumours may metastasise but do not invade adjacent tissues   T
D transcoelomic metastases are a common finding at laparotomy   F
E HRT may reasonably be prescribed after surgery for ovarian cancer   T   4.

4.19 Vesicovaginal fistulae

A the commonest cause in the UK is obstructed labour   F
B if bladder damage is recognized it should be repaired in two layers   ?   T
C free catheter drainage is essential after repair   T
D the three swab test is the best investigation to determine the site of a fistula   F
E congenital defects never occur   F

4.20   HRT

A is contraceptive in women over the age of 45 years

B should always be offered to women with premature ovarian failure

C when requested by a patient, is associated with a greater than normal incidence of psychological disorder

D should always include a progestogen for a woman with an intact uterus, to
prevent oestrogen-related endometrial hypoplasia and frank malignancy

E can be given as oestrogen alone in the woman who has undergone any
form of transcervical resection/ablation of the endometrium

4.21   Women with gestational trophoblastic disease

A are more likely to be in their 20s

B are more likely to be blood group B or AB

C may present with neurological symptoms

D are more likely to share the same blood group as their partner

E are more likely to have a balanced genetic translocation

4.22   Genital prolapse is associated with

A multiparity

B prolonged second stage of labour

C obesity

D forceps delivery

E poor nutrition

4.23   During the menopause

A plasma cholesterol, triglycerides and high density lipoproteins all rise and
very low density lipoproteins fall

B osteoporotic bones are relatively calcium depleted

C 40% of women over the age of 70 years will at some time have a fracture
of the distal radius or the femoral neck or of a vertebral body

D 15% of women who have a fracture of the femoral neck will die within a
year of the injury

E hypertensive patients or those with a history of thromboembolic disease
should not be treated with HRT

4.24 Abnormal uterine bleeding

A is commonly due to malignant cause in the postmenopausal group ? F ✓ //
B is more likely to resolve after treatment of an ectropion if the patient takes the oral contraceptive pill F
C carcinoma of the corpus uteri becomes a more likely diagnosis with increasing time from the menopause T
D carcinoma of the cervix is excluded with a recent negative smear F
E hysteroscopy/D&C may be omitted in a frail patient with obvious atrophic cervicitis T F

4

4.25 Hyperprolactinaemia is associated with

A chronic renal failure T
B galactorrhoea T F T
C cimetidine therapy F
D methyldopa therapy F T
E adrenogenital syndrome F

3

4.26 In recurrent spontaneous abortion

A the frequency of three consecutive abortions is approximately 1.6% F ?08%
B 70% of affected women will have a spontaneous resolution leading to a normal pregnancy T
C obesity and a raised mid-follicular phase LH markedly increase its incidence T
D treatment with long-acting GnRH analogues, to suppress pituitary LH, prior to gonadotrophin therapy has been successful T
E PCOS is found in 70% of cases T F

82% 4

4.27 The Fallopian tubes

A pelvic tuberculosis has a predilection for the tubes T
B tubes affected by tuberculosis are invariably occluded T F
C primary endometriosis of the tubes is common F
D there is an increased risk of ectopic pregnancy after mild tubal infection T
E surgical excision is indicated for large tubo-ovarian endometriotic lesions T

(3) T.

4

4.28 In primary infertility

A anovulation occurs in over 20% of cases T
B 1 in 10 couples exhibit difficulty in conceiving T
C a prolactin level greater than 800 mU/l can cause anovulation T
D sulphasalazine causes an increase in semen count F
E rubella immunity should be confirmed F. T

4

4.29 In contraception

A contraceptive effectiveness is expressed in the number of pregnancies per 100 women years, and is known as the Pearl Index T
B the major contraceptive action of an IUCD is to interfere with implantation of the morula F blastocyst
C the oral contraceptive pill is associated with an increase in the incidence of cervical and endometrial malignancy and a decrease in ovarian malignancy F
D the dominant mode of action of a combined oral contraceptive pill is inhibition of the mid-follicular phase LH, thus inhibiting ovulation F
E the progestogen only pill is unsuitable in the puerperium as it inhibits lactation F

4

4.30 Radiotherapy in gynaecology

A brachytherapy is the primary method of irradiation after surgery for carcinoma of the cervix
B radical radiotherapy is the treatment of choice in stage 1 vaginal cancer
C with the advent of cytotoxic chemotherapy, radiotherapy is rarely used in the treatment of epithelial ovarian cancer
D radiotherapy is an effective palliating agent for the pain of distant metastases
E inguinal node metastases from carcinoma of the vulva are radioresistant

4.31 Clomiphene citrate

A acts as a strong antioestrogen F T
B works directly at the level of the ovary F
C the multiple pregnancy rate is less than 2% F 6%
D yellow vision is a rare side-effect T
E cervical mucus hostility has been reported T

4

4.32 Cancer of the

A Fallopian tube characteristically presents with a thick brown vaginal discharge in postmenopausal women

B cervix may present in advanced stages with normal cytology

C Fallopian tube is best treated by systemic chemotherapy using platinum-based compounds

D vulva may arise from a premalignant lichen sclerosus lesion

E vagina has been linked with maternal administration of diethylstilboestrol during pregnancy

4.33 Regarding premalignant disease of the cervix

A HPV type 33 is associated with CIN

B dyskaryotic cells characteristically have a perinuclear halo

C a cell described as koilocytotic is in the premalignant phase

D interpretation of smears from postmenopausal women may be easier after topical oestrogen application

E established areas of CIN may occasionally be seen to regress

4.34 Hyperstimulation syndrome is associated with

A clomiphene administration

B DIC

C multiple pregnancy

D pleural effusions

E acute renal failure

4.35 Congenital anomalies of the female genital tract

A are common, being seen in 6% of the female population

B may result in the testicular feminization syndrome where the patient is phenotypically female and genotypically male

C include mixed gonadal dysgenesis where the patient may be a normal female, of intermediate sex or a normal male

D with vaginal agenesis has 40–50% association with renal tract anomalies

E with cervical atresia necessitates the formation of a fistula to gain successful pregnancies

4.36 Malignant disease of the corpus uteri

A endometrial carcinoma is the commonest gynaecological malignancy in the USA
B secondary spread of cancer to the uterine corpus is rare
C endometrial carcinoma arising in the fundus usually metastasises via lymphatics to the pelvic lymph nodes
D malignant change in a uterine fibroid leads to rhabdomyosarcoma formation
E squamous cancer of the endometrium may occur in an area of metaplastic epithelium

4.37 Menorrhagia

A is defined as a blood loss in excess of 80 ml per period
B is present in less than 20% of women between the ages of 16 and 45
C has no pathological cause in 50% of cases
D is associated with hypothyroidism
E can result from progestogen therapy

4.38 The menarche

A has six stages of breast development described
B may have a precocious onset, which is defined as onset of periods at less than 9 years of age
C is said to be delayed if there is no sign of thelarche or pubic hair by the age of 14 years
D may have a premature onset due to a malignant oestrogen-producing tumour in pseudoprecocious puberty
E is consequent upon two hypothalamic factors: pulsatile GnRH production and a decrease in the threshold of sensitivity to circulating sex steroids

4.39 Surgical complications commonly occur at the following times

A paralytic ileus at 7 days
B atelectasis in the first 24 hours
C wound dehiscence in the second week
D secondary haemorrhage at 10–14 days
E deep venous thrombosis in the first 2 days

4.40   Endometrial resection

A should be performed in patients suffering with purely menorrhagia

B sterility is assured

C uterus should not be retroverted

D pretreatment with danazol is necessary

E when performed in the luteal phase is most successful

4.41   The menstrual cycle

A begins with each ovary containing approximately 100 000 primordial follicles

B is usually characterized with a dominant follicle at ovulation measuring 20 mm ± 3 mm

C is associated with follicles comprising a polar body and a cumulus oophorus surrounded by the zona pellucida and the corona radiata

D commences with each primordial follicle having an oocyte arrested in mitotic prophase

E may lead to a luteotrophic corpus luteum which will degenerate to a corpus albicans with time

4.42   Cancer of the cervix

A affects 2000 women in England and Wales annually

B is associated with infection with human papilloma virus types 6 and 8

C occurs more frequently in smokers of higher social class

D has a peak age of incidence in the seventh decade of life

E is more likely to be an adenocarcinoma in the younger age group

4.43   The following can be performed using the laparoscope

A enucleation of subserosal fibroids

B adhesiolysis

C hysterectomy

D enterocele repair

E appendicectomy

4.44 During the neonatal, infant and childhood years of a female

A there is a relative lack of oestrogen leading to a prominent clitoris and vestibule
B a positive culture of *Neisseria gonorrhoea* implies some kind of sexual contact in the first instance, if the mother is seronegative
C a positive chlamydia culture is best treated with tetracyclines
D a sterile round vulval ulcer with a granular base is usually benign
E sarcoma botryoides is best treated by a Wertheim's hysterectomy with a total vaginectomy

4.45 Secondary amenorrhoea

A occurs after 6 months in the absence of a physiological cause or hysterectomy
B in association with cyclic pelvic pain suggests an iatrogenic cause
C of adrenal origin may be associated with galactorrhoea
D is more likely in long-distance runners than javelin throwers
E when stress-related is best treated by oral contraceptive therapy

4.46 Pelvic pain

A occurs in over 30% of gynaecological outpatient referrals
B Crohn's disease is part of the differential diagnosis
C laparoscopy is the investigation of choice
D transuterine venography has been used
E transvaginal ultrasound can be used to delineate masses

4.47 In USS

A Professor Ian Donald pioneered the technique in obstetrics and gynaecology in the 1950s
B the vibrations propagate through the medium as a pulsed sinusoidal wave with amplitude, frequency and wavelength
C transvaginal scanning is more accurate than transabdominal in the initial assessment of gynaecological disorders
D if the signal is transmitted along the axis of a blood vessel then the magnitude of the red blood cells in the vessel can be related to the shift in Doppler frequency
E an ectopic pregnancy can always be diagnosed before surgery

4.48 Carcinoma of the vulva

A cure rates are significantly higher if radical excision is accompanied by bilateral inguinal node dissection T

B the triple incision procedure is contraindicated in the presence of large matted and fixed inguinal lymph nodes

C the incidence of chronic lymphoedema of the lower limbs may be reduced by suction drainage of groin wounds

D local treatment is sufficient for microinvasive disease less than 5 mm beneath the basement membrane

E radical surgery is often recommended for palliation in the frail and very old patients

4.49 Polycystic ovary syndrome

A occurs in over 20% of women F T

B is associated with hirsutism T

C is found in 5% of infertile patients T

D results in enlarged ovaries T

E is associated with a decrease in luteinizing hormone F   4

4.50 In sexual physiology

A the plateau phase succeeds orgasm

B up to 50% of male erectile problems may be due to psychological causes

C the male orgasm is necessary for fertilization to occur

D intact functioning spinal cord centres at T11–12 and S2–4 are necessary for full sexual enjoyment

E in the male, vasodilation and engorgement of the corpora cavernosa results in an erection

4.51 Germ cell tumours of the ovary

A generally affect younger women more than their epithelial counterparts T

B usually respond well to cytotoxic chemotherapy T

C a struma ovarii is a monophyletic germ cell tumour comprising functional thyroid tissue T

D dysgerminoma is a malignant tumour of primordial germ cell origin and has a 5-year survival greater than 90% T

E single-agent chemotherapy with a platinum-based analogue is the commonest therapy in the UK F

S

4.52 Premenstrual syndrome

A only 2% of women are severely affected   T

B symptoms can occur throughout the cycle   F

C caused by progesterone deficiency   F

D associated with loss of libido   T

E cured by hysterectomy and bilateral salpingo-oophorectomy   T

S

4.53 In the female genitalia

A the clitoris is anatomically similar to the penis in that it has three crura   F

B the remnants of the hymen are known as the carunculae myrtiformes   T

C the neonatal uterus decreases in size after birth by up to one-third   T

D the vaginal glands secrete fluids during sexual arousal   T   F

E 10% of women of reproductive age have a retroflexed and retroverted uterus   T   ?

4.54 Common associations in pelvic inflammatory disease are

A acute PID and *Mycobacterium tuberculosis*   T   F

B deep dyspareunia and acute PID   T   F

C *Actinomyces israelii* and an IUCD   T

D perihepatic adhesions and chlamydia infection   T   F   T

E beta-haemolytic streptococci and postpartum infection   T

3.

4.55 The following are associated with ectopic pregnancy

A exposure to diethylstilboestrol *in utero*   F   T

B sterilization   T

C retroversion of the uterus   F

D women under 18   F

E chlamydial infection in the pelvis   T

4

4.56 In the anatomy of the pelvis

A the somatic nerve lumbar plexus is formed by branches of T12, L1–L4

B the femoral nerves arises from the second, third and fourth lumbar nerves

C the common iliac lymph nodes are usually arranged in medial, lateral and posterior chains around the common iliac artery

D transection of the inferior mesenteric artery will lead to ischaemia of the lower bowel

E the levator ani can be divided into three components—puborectalis, pubo-coccygeus and iliococcygeus

4.57 Radiotherapy

A the SI (Systeme Internationale) unit of dosage of ionising radiation is the Rad

B sensitivity to ionising radiation increases in the hypoxic cell

C modern high-energy external beam machines have the advantage of delivering maximum dose at a greater depth

D cell death occurs more readily in rapidly dividing cell populations due to disruption of cell metabolism

E caesium-137 is a commonly used brachytherapy source

4.58 The following can result in anovulation

A progesterone-only contraception T (?) what about depo provera.

B acromegaly T

C hyperthyroidism T

D PCOS T

E diabetes mellitus T. F

4.59 In the human

A the hypothalamus lies between the optic chiasm and the mammillary bodies

B the anterior pituitary gland does not receive an arterial blood supply

C LHRH will stimulate production of FSH as well as LH T

D serotonin will predominantly stimulate release of gonadotrophins T

E in PCOS there is a reversed FSH:LH ratio of approximately 3:1 F

LH T

4.60 Accepted parameters for a normal semen analysis are

A a sperm count of 10–20 million per ml F

B a volume of 1 ml F

C 60% motility T

D 60% abnormal forms F

E a positive mixed agglutination reaction F

PRACTICE PAPER FIVE

Allow 1 hour for the completion of all 60 questions

Answers are on p. 127

5.1 The following statements concern hysterectomies

A over 90% of patients are satisfied with the operation
B the mortality rate following a hysterectomy is 1 in 10 000 patients
C ovarian removal is always performed during an abdominal hysterectomy
D the size of fibroids determines the route of hysterectomy
E previous Caesarean section contraindicates vaginal hysterectomy

5.2 In urethral sphincter dysfunction

A a plain anteroposterior X-ray will reveal a full bladder associated with chronic retention of urine
B childbirth may be responsible for denervation of the sphincter mechanisms
C 6 months of pelvic floor physiotherapy will improve symptoms in 70% of women awaiting surgery
D only 40% of women using vaginal cones will be cured or improved
E anterior colporrhaphy will improve the condition of urinary incontinence when associated with detrusor instability

5.3 Carcinoma of the vagina

A comprises 10% of female genital malignancies
B involvement of the lower vagina leads to inguinal node metastases
C clear cell carcinoma may occur in patients who took stilboestrol in pregnancy
D many patients who present post-hysterectomy have a history of CIN
E the risk of developing carcinoma of the vagina should be considered in patients who require long-term vaginal pessaries for prolapse

5.4 Septic abortion

A is associated with criminal abortions
B must be treated with intravenous antibiotics prior to evacuation
C is commonly due to infection after an incomplete abortion
D can present with pyrexia, pain and bleeding
E is associated with uterine congenital anomalies

5.5 In urinary incontinence surgery

A vaginal capacity and mobility do not need assessing before colposuspension

B an artificial urinary sphincter is indicated when conventional surgery has failed and the options of continual incontinence, catheter drainage or urinary diversion are unacceptable

C postoperative residual urinary volumes should be less than 50 ml on at least three occasions before removal of a suprapubic catheter

D 10% of women who undergo a Marshall–Marchetti–Krantz procedure suffer from postoperative osteitis pubis

E cystoscopy is not always necessary following endoscopic bladder neck suspension operations

5.6 Sexually transmitted diseases

A a rash often accompanies primary syphilis

B the VDRL test measures antibody to treponemal cardiolipin antigen

C a gumma is the term applied to chronic lesions of tertiary syphilis

D penicillin is no longer the first-line antibiotic in active syphilis

E screening for syphilis in pregnancy is by the VDRL and TPHA tests

5.7 Recurrent spontaneous abortion

A is defined as three consecutive abortions

B has a frequency of approximately 8%

C over 80% of patients will attain a pregnancy with just psychological support

D a raised day 8 LH level greater than 10 IU/l increases the miscarriage risk

E PCOS is less common in recurrent aborters

5.8 In definitive contraception with sterilization

A female sterilization is surgically safer than male sterilization

B after vasectomy, recanalization of the vas occurs in 1–4:10 000 cases

C women under the age of 25 years should never be offered sterilization

D female reversal of sterilization shows a successful pregnancy rate of 70%

E it may lead to antisperm antibodies in men after vasectomy

5.9 Endometriosis

A invariably occurs if there is retrograde menstruation
B is associated with an increased volume of free fluid in the peritoneal cavity
C is frequently asymptomatic
D may be treated by progestogens such as gestrinone
E patients successfully treated by medical therapy have a 20% chance of recurrence by 2 years

5.10 Bartholin's glands

A can commonly be infected by *E. coli*
B are remnants of mesonephric origin
C are situated posteriorly to Skene's duct cysts
D should be marsupialized when acutely infected
E carcinoma can occur within the gland and has a less favourable prognosis than squamous cell carcinoma of the vulva

5.11 During the menopause

A 25% of women have hot flushes and night sweats for 5 years
B head, axillary and pubic hair is lost whilst facial hair may increase
C plasma cholesterol, HDL and triglycerides all rise, thus leading to an increase in ischaemic heart disease in this age group
D the characteristic symptoms of vasomotor instability, anxiety and difficulty in concentration may mimic a carcinoid tumour
E the administration of oestrogen-containing HRT will reverse the associated osteoporosis

5.12 Regarding subfertile males

A a history of urological surgery may suggest retrograde ejaculation
B azoospermia suggesting a mechanical blockage may be investigated by operative vasography
C oligospermia is present with a sperm count of 50 million or less per ml of semen
D in unexplained oligospermia good results are obtained with clomiphene
E direct injection of sperm into the ovum using a micropipette has been used for men with abnormal sperm morphology

5.13   Deep dyspareunia can be caused by

A Bartholin's cyst
B appendicitis
C psychosexual problems
D adenomyosis
E fibroids

5.14   During the menstrual cycle

A early follicular phase FSH rises lead to granulosa cell oestradiol production
B menstrual blood loss is 50% venous and 50% arterial
C spiral arterioles and basal arterioles are very influenced by the changing hormonal milieu of the luteal phase of the cycle
D luteal phase endometrium forms lipid- and glycogen-rich subnuclear vacuoles 48 hours after ovulation
E granulocyte and lymphocyte infiltration of the endometrial stroma is seen

5.15   Malignancy in the vagina

A squamous cell carcinoma of the vault metastasises primarily via blood-borne emboli to the liver
B the commonest presenting symptom is abnormal bleeding
C radiotherapy is the treatment of choice for stage II disease
D sarcoma botryoides is a tumour commonly found in the elderly
E the incidence of clear cell carcinoma is likely to rise in the next century

5.16   Ectopic pregnancy

A over 80% of patients present with pain and amenorrhoea
B over 75% of patients will experience abnormal vaginal bleeding
C pain always precedes the abnormal vaginal bleeding
D abdominal ultrasound is the investigation of choice
E more common in women over 35 years of age

5.17 In radiology

A an IVU is mandatory in FIGO staging of a cervical carcinoma

B the principle of MRI depends upon the absorption then re-emission of radio energy after certain nuclei are placed within a magnetic field and stimulated by radio waves

C the female pelvis is particularly suited to MRI as it is relatively unaffected by cardiac motion

D CT can be safely used in those patients with a hip prosthesis

E a recent myocardial infarction is not a contraindication to MRI

5.18 Premalignant disease of the cervix

A a dilute vinegar solution is used in diagnosis

B an area of raised epithelium with large irregular vessels is suggestive of microinvasive disease

C the treatment of choice is large loop diathermy excision

D koilocytosis and dyskaryosis may be observed on the same slide; both have a viral aetiology

E satellite lesions on colposcopy suggest viral infection not leading to intraepithelial neoplasia

5.19 The following concern leiomyomata

A diagnosis is always possible using ultrasound

B myomectomy is advocated in women wishing to conserve fertility

C GnRH agonists are used to decrease size and also blood loss at operation

D submucous leiomyomata cause menorrhagia and impaired implantation

E the use of the combined oral contraceptive pill protects against development of leiomyomata

5.20 In evaluation of a woman with a urinary problem

A cystometry is performed to calculate the intravesical volume during different urinary states

B the detrusor pressure in a normal female is said to be less than 20 cmH$_2$O

C a flow rate of 10 ml/s may be due to previous bladder neck surgery

D spontaneous voiding followed by catheterization which reveals a residual of 50% of normal bladder capacity may lead to a diagnosis of chronic urinary retention

E neurophysiological testing of L2–L4 may be useful to assess the bladder

5.21 Malignancy of the corpus uteri

A is less common in the nulliparous patient
B less than 5% of cases occur in the premenopausal patient
C it is unusual for a sarcoma to arise in a pre-existing fibroid
D endometrial carcinoma is staged at laparotomy
E early lymphatic spread from a carcinoma of the fundus is to the para-aortic nodes

5.22 Ureteric injury

A transection can occur during abdominal hysterectomy
B repair of transection over a stent with an absorbable suture is normal
C a Boari flap is used to repair a ureterovaginal fistula
D obstruction may require reimplantation
E unrecognized transection can present with peritonitis

5.23 In female congenital anomalies

A the Frank's procedure is the treatment of choice in all cases of congenital absence of the vagina and uterus
B an absent cervix in the presence of a functional uterus is not uncommon
C the mesonephric ducts may migrate and fuse in an anomalous way to form a uterus didelphys
D diethylstilboestrol has been implicated
E a deficiency of the adrenal enzyme, 11-hydroxylase is the commonest cause of congenital adrenal hyperplasia

5.24 Complications of gynaecological surgery

A the shocked patient in the immediate postoperative period must be assumed to be bleeding from the operation site unless otherwise indicated
B collapse of a segment of lung in the first 24 hours is termed atelectasis and warrants prompt antibiotic treatment
C large-volume blood transfusion predisposes to ARDS
D localized wound infection should be treated with a broad-spectrum anti-biotic
E urinary tract injury should always be treated by early surgical repair

5.25   The following concern genital prolapse

A vault prolapse follows 5% of vaginal hysterectomy
B the majority of patients are asymptomatic
C coital difficulties can be common
D squamous cell carcinoma can occur
E the use of HRT at the menopause should be encouraged

5.26   In genetic studies it has been found that

A the majority of ovarian cancers are aneuploid
B there is a strong link between borderline ovarian tumours and trisomy 12
C if the number of sex chromosomes increases beyond three, there is a strong
   tendency to mental retardation
D the 45X chromosome constitution has an overall incidence of 1:5000 live
   births
E XXX females have an increased incidence of psychosis and short stature

5.27   Ovarian cancer

A Brenner tumours are epithelial in origin and resemble urothelium on histology
B CA 125 is often elevated in stromal cell ovarian malignances
C *Pseudomyxoma peritonei* is more commonly related to benign than malignant ovarian tumours
D carboplatin is the chemotherapeutic agent of choice for epithelial ovarian
   cancer in most units
E there is currently an effective screening programme for familial ovarian
   cancer

5.28   The following concern hyperprolactinaemia

A pituitary adenoma is present in only 25% of cases
B PCOS commonly coexists
C the drug of choice is methyldopa
D prolactin levels over 600 mU/l are diagnostic
E primary hypothyroidism occurs in 25% of cases

5.29   In minimally invasive surgery

A the risk of fluid overload with pulmonary and cerebral oedema is of the order of 5%
B during hysteroscopy the maximum flow rate of CO_2 is 100 ml/min
C endometrial resection results in 70% amenorrhoea rates
D it is true that techniques available are only used for benign pathology
E acute pelvic sepsis is a contraindication to hysteroscopy

5.30   Gestational trophoblastic disease

A hydatidiform moles arise from paternal genetic material
B choriocarcinoma is characterized by an absence of chorionic villi
C there is a high incidence in South-East Asia
D choriocarcinoma is highly chemosensitive with methotrexate as the agent most frequently used
E over 80% of patients with hydatidiform mole have beta-hCG levels that return to normal by 8 weeks after suction evacuation

5.31   Infertility

A a day 21 progesterone over 10 nmol/l confirms ovulation
B a D&C is essential in assessment
C a PCT is important in assessing sperm mucus interaction and can be performed at any stage in the cycle
D basal body temperature charts show a 3°C rise at mid-cycle to suggest ovulation
E hypothyroidism can cause anovulation

5.32   In the female breast

A a cystosarcoma phylloides may be benign
B a large dose of radiation is used during mammography
C galactorrhoea is a common presentation in hyperprolactinaemia
D development of a breast cancer during pregnancy is associated with an increased 5-year mortality
E lactation can occur from an accessory breast

5.33 Cervical cancer

A there is an association between HPV infection and the development of adenocarcinoma
B cancers in elderly women are more likely to be adenocarcinomata
C it is highly unusual for squamous and glandular malignant tissue to arise in the same tumour
D lymph node metastases occur in less than 1% of stage I tumours
E the majority of recurrences occur between 3 and 5 years after primary treatment

5.34 Management of anovulation

A clomiphene treatment can result in an increased abortion rate
B tamoxifen can be used
C cyclofenil is thought to enhance production of oestrogenic mucus
D human menopausal gonadotrophin (hMG) treatment can result in a 60% multiple pregnancy rate
E hMG can result in hyperstimulation syndrome in 20% of cases

5.35 In infertility management

A the female mid-cycle temperature rise of 0.5–1.0°C is due to the thermogenic effects of progesterone
B a postcoital test is best performed in the immediate postovulatory phase of the menstrual cycle
C the mixed antiglobulin reaction is useful in assessing cervical mucus antigenicity
D it is known that the first part of the male seminal ejaculate contains the highest number of sperm
E for a male with a sperm count of less than 20 million/ml the overall pregnancy rate without therapy is approximately 50%

5.36 Vulval dystrophy

A has a multifactorial aetiology
B steroid creams are the mainstay of treatment
C there is an inflammatory infiltrate in the superficial skin layers
D there are often features of skin trauma which are self-inflicted
E there is invariably a loss of rete ridges on histological examination of a skin biopsy

5.37 IVF is associated with

A pelvic abscess
B a cumulative success rate of 60% after 2 cycles
C ectopic pregnancy
D intrauterine growth retardation
E premature delivery

5.38 In disorders of puberty

A impaired olfactory sensation and delayed pubertal development are more common in girls than in boys
B a craniopharyngioma may result in primary amenorrhoea and oestrogen deficiency
C a critical fat:lean muscle mass ratio of at least 20% is necessary for menarche to occur
D histiocytosis-X in children leading to delayed growth and puberty is known as Hand–Schuller–Christian disease
E primary amenorrhoea is defined as the failure to menstruate by the age of 18 years

5.39 Radiotherapy

A ionising radiation injures the genetic apparatus of the dividing cell
B adjuvant radiotherapy is commonly administered for lymph node metastases in cervical, uterine and ovarian cancer
C anaemia is a frequent side-effect due to cell death in the bone marrow
D results in early-stage cervical cancer are similar to those of surgery
E an afterloading machine delivers external beam therapy to the patient

5.40 Dysfunctional uterine bleeding

A is associated with anticoagulant therapy
B results in 50% of women with menorrhagia
C can cause menstrual blood loss in excess of 200 ml
D is associated with endometriosis
E can be treated successfully with ethamsylate

5.41 The Fallopian tubes

A show characteristic diverticulae at hysterosalpingography in salpingitis isthmica nodosa

B are responsible for 50% of female infertility

C with salpingitis and the liver with perihepatic adhesions are linked in the Fitz–Hugh–Curtis syndrome

D are best sutured with fine absorbable suture material to prevent adhesion formation

E when damaged by tuberculosis are best treated by medical methods, not surgical

5.42 Genital herpes

A the likely infecting agent is herpes simplex type 1

B herpes simplex is an RNA virus

C treatment should be deferred until the diagnosis is confirmed by laboratory investigation

D latent virus resides in the sacral ganglia

E menstruation may be a stimulus for a recurrent attack

5.43 Management of menorrhagia

A mefenamic acid can result in a decrease in blood loss of up to 30%

B tranexamic acid is contraindicated when low levels of antithrombin III are present

C medical treatment is successful in over 80% of cases

D danazol treatment can result in permanent voice changes

E a D&C is successful treatment in 50% of cases

5.44 In ectopic pregnancy

A cervical ectopic pregnancy has an incidence of 1:25 000

B any form of contraception is associated with a decreased incidence compared with non-users of contraception

C prior exposure to diethylstilboestrol is linked with an increased incidence

D the Arias-Stella phenomenon is diagnostic

E the major complication is death

5.45 Amenorrhoea

A postpill amenorrhoea is associated with high gonadotrophin levels
B associated tunnel vision suggests a hypothalamic tumour
C a short patient with absent secondary sexual characteristics should have karyotyping to exclude Klinefelter's syndrome
D there is often a family history in those with premature menopause
E tumours of the posterior pituitary if hormone-secreting may present with galactorrhoea

5.46 Endometrial resection

A should be performed when the family is complete
B perforation should be followed by laparotomy
C pretreatment with danazol is essential
D submucous fibroids are a contraindication
E adenomyosis often results in failure

5.47 An IUCD

A is more likely to perforate the uterus or be expelled from the uterus if inserted earlier than 6 weeks postnatally
B carries an increased risk of complications if inserted into a woman who has undergone a Caesarean section in the past 3 months
C when *in situ*, is associated with an ectopic pregnancy rate of up to 9%
D can be safely left in the uterus for at least 5 years without lowering efficacy
E is absolutely contraindicated in any woman with a history of a sexually transmitted disease in the past 12 months

5.48 Known pathogens in pelvic inflammatory disease include

A *Neisseria gonorrhoea*—a gram-negative diplococcus
B the bacteroides species—facultative aerobes
C *Mycoplasma hominis*
D beta-haemolytic streptococci—gram-negative cocci
E *Escherichia coli*—a gram-negative rod

5.49 The following can result in pelvic pain

A endometriosis
B PCOS
C pelvic venous congestion
D porphyria
E shingles

5.50 In the human female

A only 5% of women are completely free from premenstrual symptoms
B the diuretic spironolactone can be used in the treatment of hirsutism
C 5% of women with PCOS also have hyperprolactinaemia
D a normal urinary 17-ketosteroid excretion rate excludes the presence of a virilizing adrenal tumour
E the SHBG is raised if she is on an oestrogen-containing oral contraceptive pill

5.51 Non-epithelial tumours of the ovary

A tumours arising from sex cord and other stromal elements commonly have a predominantly cystic component
B Meig's syndrome occurs in association with a fibrosarcoma
C adult granulosa cell tumours are generally of low-grade malignancy
D androblastomata differentiate into Sertoli and Leydig cell types
E stromal cell tumours are markedly chemosensitive

5.52 The following are associated with polycystic ovary syndrome

A decreased level of androstenedione
B raised oestrone
C reversed LH:FSH ratio of 3:1
D enlarged almond-shaped ovaries
E necklace of small follicles all less than 5 mm diameter

5.53 In the human female

A vaginal and urethral epithelia have the highest concentrations of oestrogen receptors in the body

B there is a 30% loss of skin collagen in the first 10 years after the menopause

C premature ovarian failure affects 1% of women less than 40 years of age

D oestradiol is the major oestrogen produced by the postmenopausal woman

E a standard 1.25 mg dose of vaginal conjugated oestrogen cream will achieve a higher plasma level of oestradiol than that produced by the same dose given orally

5.54 Investigation of abnormal uterine bleeding

A a cervical smear should be deferred in the presence of active bleeding and the patient told to return for examination after the bleeding has ceased

B a failed attempt at aspiration histology of the uterine cavity due to a stenosed os in a postmenopausal patient suggests atrophic vaginitis as a cause and local oestrogen therapy is warranted

C aspiration histology of the uterine cavity is likely to provide a sample of endometrium comparable to that obtained at D&C

D if a patient re-bleeds 7 months after thorough investigation has led to a diagnosis of atrophic vaginitis it is reasonable to treat her with oestrogen cream

E hysteroscopy may be possible under local anaesthesia in the outpatient clinic

5.55 Management of PMS

A placebo response is in excess of 60%

B pyridoxine treatment can result in a peripheral neuropathy

C linoleic acid administration results in an enhanced response to ß-endorphin

D oestrogen therapy has been shown to be better than placebo

E progestogen therapy can result in worsening symptoms

5.56 In the human male

A testicular interstitial Leydig cells produce testosterone

B accessory gland secretions constitute at least 90% of the seminal volume

C karyotypically abnormal males with azoospermia are predominantly 47 XXY

D erectile and ejaculatory failure may be caused by chronic renal failure

E approximately 1% of ejaculated sperm reach the Fallopian tubes

5.57 Regarding choriocarcinoma

A single-agent chemotherapy with methotrexate is used in high-risk disease
B adjuvant radiotherapy is commonly used in high-risk disease
C surgical excision of chemoresistant metastases improves prognosis
D the tumour marker beta-hCG is the most sensitive monitor of response
E fertility rates after successful treatment exceed 60%

5.58 The following can result in genital prolapse

A nulliparity
B spina bifida
C prolonged second stage
D ascites
E smoking

5.59 The ovary

A receives its arterial supply from vessels arising from the aorta just above the origin of the renal arteries
B may undergo malignant change in Sertoli–Leydig cell tumours
C is best imaged by CT or MRI rather than USS
D is best removed via a longitudinal abdominal incision in cases of suspected malignancy
E in malignant disease can be accurately assessed by using CA 125 as a marker

5.60 Cervical cancer

A small cell non-keratinizing squamous cell cancer has a relatively good prognosis
B cystoscopy may be omitted when staging posterior cervical tumours
C 5-year survival rates of around 50% may be achieved after pelvic exenteration for recurrent cancer
D squamous cancer is not responsive to chemotherapy
E 5-year survival in stage I disease with positive pelvic lymph nodes is around 60%

PRACTICE PAPER SIX

Allow 1 hour for the completion of all 60 questions

Answers are on p. 135

6.1 The following are associated with spontaneous abortions

A presence of lupus anticoagulant
B family history of spontaneous abortion
C cervical incompetence
D *Candida* infection
E PCOS

6.2 In the neuropathic bladder patient

A the bowel, lower limbs and sexual function are also usually affected
B the best form of screening the whole urinary tract is a micturating cysto-urethrogram
C contractile dysfunction may be treated with an augmentation 'clam' duode-nocystoplasty
D the majority of lesions distal to the sacral parasympathetic outflow are due to diabetes and trauma
E the bladder may become so thick-walled it occludes the ureters in their intramural portion leading to vesicoureteric junction obstruction

6.3 In menopause

A urinary frequency may be related to a local oestrogen deficiency
B calcium supplements are as effective as oestrogen therapy in preventing osteoporosis provided bone mass is normal
C testosterone may be added to the HRT regimen if loss of libido is a symp-tom
D there is gradual loss of total body hair
E there is a rise in HDL levels, predisposing to ischaemic heart disease

6.4   Superficial dyspareunia can be caused by

A   vulval dystrophy
B   episiotomy repair
C   retroverted uterus
D   ovarian cyst
E   inflammatory bowel disease

6.5   In the female

A   voiding three times at night is normal
B   50% will develop a UTI at some time during their life
C   up to 30% of women with asymptomatic bacteriuria develop acute pyelonephritis in pregnancy
D   urinary tract schistosomiasis will usually cause an eosinophilia
E   with recurrent UTIs, management will include drinking at least 2 litres of fluid per day and prompt voiding after intercourse

6.6   Regarding the Fallopian tubes

A   purulent infection in the tubes leads to a hydrosalpinx
B   pelvic clearance is recommended for tuberculous salpingitis
C   malignant change is rare with less than 100 cases of primary carcinoma per year
D   Fallopian tube cancer has a predilection for spread to the omentum
E   chemotherapy is rarely used in treatment of tubal malignancy

6.7   Ectopic pregnancy

A   occurs in approximately 1 in 130 births in the UK
B   the commonest site for an ectopic pregnancy is in the ampulla of the tube
C   cervical ectopics often require tamponade with a Foley catheter
D   has been treated conservatively with methotrexate
E   the risk of recurrence is less than 10%

6.8 The urinary bladder

A fundus can communicate with the umbilicus via the urachal remnants, the median umbilical ligaments

B has a trigone delineated by the two ureteric orifices and the external urethral orifice

C in the adult male has a mean volume of 220 ml, with a range of 120–320 ml

D is innervated by spinal cord segments T11–L1 and S2–S4

E in the female is connected to the 6 cm long, 4 mm wide urethra

6.9 A patient with carcinoma of the corpus uteri

A has a 25% risk of dying of the disease

B has a 15% chance of a family history of the disease

C is likely to have been prescribed beta-blocking drugs

D is less likely to have had children

E may have been taking Premarin tablets

6.10 Management of fibroids

A abdominal hysterectomy is the usual treatment

B myomectomy has a recurrence rate of 10%

C HRT is contraindicated in the presence of fibroids

D fibroids regrow on cessation of GnRH therapy

E vasopressin is contraindicated

6.11 In the vulva

A lichen sclerosus is a premalignant condition

B intertrigo is often associated with a candidal infection

C the vulva is affected in Crohn's disease in 25–30% of cases

D cysts on the anterior vulva can arise from peritoneum associated with the round ligament

E condyloma acuminata are mostly due to HPV subtypes 7 and 11

6.12   Premalignant disease of the cervix

A Lugol's iodine is commonly applied and demonstrates colposcopic features of CIN such as mosaicism

B coarse punctation is associated with severe dyskaryosis

C squamous metaplasia may exhibit acetowhite change which may be confused with premalignant disease

D CIN is very unlikely to involve gland crypts

E laser cone biopsy is more precise and gives a superior surgical specimen for histological analysis as compared to LLETZ

6.13   Fistulae in obstetrics and gynaecology

A continuous incontinence along with voluntary micturition is a result of a small vesicovaginal fistula

B CPD is the commonest cause of a vesicovaginal fistula in the third world

C a low fistula is repaired by a combined vaginal and abdominal approach

D radiotherapy is a common cause

E in a high fistula a micturating cystogram and an IVU should be performed

6.14   In the assessment of female urinary function

A it is known that up to 30% of young healthy nulliparous females are occasionally incontinent of urine

B GSI can be diagnosed on symptoms alone

C detrusor instability may be present in multiple sclerosis

D phenoxybenzamine is a useful agent in treating detrusor sphincter dyssynergia

E intravaginal prostaglandins are beneficial in restoring normal bladder function after vaginal hysterectomy

6.15   The Fallopian tubes

A chronic pelvic infection affecting the tubes is likely to be due to the tubercle bacillus

B caseation is a feature of a chronic pyosalpinx after the acute phase

C squamous carcinoma is the commonest primary malignancy

D radiotherapy is commonly used to treat Fallopian tube cancer

E Fallopian tube cancer may present early with watery vaginal bleeding

6.16 Genital prolapse

A postnatal physiotherapy should be encouraged
B the use of preoperative vaginal preparations should be avoided
C a shelf pessary is best used in procidentia
D a Manchester repair is the treatment of choice if fertility is to be maintained
E posthysterectomy vaginal vault prolapse occurs in less than 2% of cases

6.17 Hormonal systems include

A the endocrine mechanism which involves glandular secretion of a regulatory substance into a circulation leading to a specific effect on another gland or structure
B glycoproteins like LH, TSH and beta-hCG
C trophic hormones which typically require 10% receptor occupation before action is evident
D adenylate cyclase and cAMP as second messengers to amplify the original small hormone signal
E maintenance of biological activity only while the nuclear site is occupied with the hormone–receptor complex

6.18 Endometrial carcinoma

A is a disease of developing countries
B malignant squamous and glandular elements may coexist
C blood-borne deposits in the liver are an early manifestation of metastatic disease
D stage I disease with invasion of less than half the myometrial thickness and a high-grade tumour is treated by hysterectomy alone
E chemotherapy for advanced disease is associated with poor survival rates

6.19 Prolactin

A gamma-aminobutyric acid release increases prolactin release
B bromocriptine is the drug of choice in hyperprolactinaemia
C is secreted from the posterior pituitary gland
D approximately one-third of patients with a microadenoma undergo spontaneous resolution
E bromocriptine should be stopped when pregnant

6.20 In assisted conception medicine

A clomiphene citrate and cyclofenil are used for their antioestrogen action
B ovulation induction with FSH alone yields significantly superior results than with human menopausal gonadotrophins
C in hypogonadotrophic hypogonadism with low LH levels, luteal support with GnRH is necessary after ovulation
D in male factor infertility, sperm density and motility are the two most important criteria for successful IVF
E legal guidelines are laid down in The Human Fertilisation and Embryology Act

6.21 Endometriosis

A is commoner in black women
B is never seen after the menopause
C it is reasonable to prescribe HRT in women treated with GnRH analogues
D it is postulated that infertility is related to phagocytosis of sperm by macrophages found in peritoneal fluid
E minimal endometriosis should always be treated due to the associated infertility

6.22 Infertility

A a prolactin level over 400 mU/l is associated with anovulation
B 15% of cases are still unexplained
C male factor infertility is increasing
D FSH/LH levels should be taken in the second half of the cycle
E fibroids do not cause infertility

6.23 In contraception

A the 'morning after pill' regimen must be given within 72 hours of unprotected intercourse
B there is no delay in return to fertility after cessation of oral progestogen-only pill contraception
C sterilization of either partner is the most widely used single form of contraception in the world
D 50–60% of men who have undergone vasectomy develop some form of sperm antibodies
E in an epileptic on phenytoin a medium-dose combined oral contraceptive pill is necessary rather than a low-dose pill

6.24 Cancer of the cervix

A para-aortic lymph node dissection is a standard part of a Wertheim hysterectomy
B a patient who presents with metastatic disease in the supraclavicular lymph nodes should be treated with chemotherapy
C over 60% of recurrences occur in the first year after primary treatment
D further radiotherapy is recommended for a central pelvic recurrence in a previously irradiated patient
E combination chemotherapy significantly increases survival rates in patients with pelvic lymph node metastases

6.25 hMG is associated with

A a decreased rate of abortion
B an increased rate of stillbirth
C multiple pregnancy in up to 30% of cases
D severe hyperstimulation syndrome in less than 1% of cases
E LHRH used at mid-cycle to facilitate ovulation

6.26 In the woman with uterine fibroids

A hyaline change is the commonest form of degeneration seen
B the risk of sarcomatous change is of the order of 0.1%
C there is a 15% association with infertility
D USS is always necessary to help confirm the nature of the mass
E a Bonney hood may be useful in their surgical management

6.27 Sexually transmitted disease

A yaws causes genital ulceration and the causative organism is an intracellular parasite
B snail track ulceration is a mucosal manifestation of secondary syphilis
C gonorrhoea rarely affects the rectum
D gonococcal arthritis is usually monoarticular
E there are many subtypes of *Chlamydia trachomatis*; types L1, L2 and L3 cause urogenital infection

6.28 Menorrhagia can be associated with

A subserous fibroids
B hyperthyroidism
C intrauterine contraceptive device
D combined oral contraceptive pill
E carcinoma of the cervix

6.29 In the abdominopelvic cavity

A the sigmoid colon lies in the lesser pelvis anterior to the broad ligament
B the ureter travels retroperitoneally along psoas major and is crossed by the gonadal vessels
C the inferior mesenteric artery arises 3–4 cm above the aortic bifurcation and ends as the superior rectal artery
D the rectum has a mesentery and appendices epiploicae
E the bladder is completely covered by peritoneum superiorly

6.30 Ovarian cancer

A patients with two relatives with ovarian cancer should be offered screening as part of a national assessment of ovarian cancer screening
B mucinous tumours are said to have differentiated along similar lines to endocervical glandular epithelium
C the oral contraceptive pill has a protective effect
D the omentum should be excised in all cases even when macroscopically normal
E bowel involvement at laparotomy should be treated with primary chemotherapy and interval debulking surgery

6.31 Surgical management of menorrhagia

A laser ablation and endometrial resection have similar success rates
B water intoxication has followed endometrial resection
C radiofrequency-induced thermal ablation can result in fistula formation
D the presence of fibroids is a contraindication to ablative therapy
E endometrial resection during the proliferative phase is essential

6.32 In the lower renal tract

A the detrusor muscle contracts as a single syncytial mass
B the pubourethral ligaments contain fibres histologically identical to the detrusor muscle
C cell bodies in sacral segments S2–4 give rise to cholinergic parasympathetic fibres to the detrusor
D active elastic tension is the most important factor leading to closure of the bladder neck sphincter and the proximal urethra
E the first desire to void urine is normally felt at half the final bladder capacity

6.33 The menopause

A hot flushes of the climacteric may last for 5 years in 25% of patients
B the ankle is a common site of osteoporotic fractures
C carcinoid syndrome gives rise to symptoms which may be erroneously attributed to the climacteric
D there is a slight increase in the incidence of thromboembolic disease in women given natural oestrogen by the transdermal route
E the advantage of oral therapy is that the 'first pass' effect due to hepatic metabolism is avoided

6.34 Hysteroscopic surgery

A endometrial resection can be performed as a day case
B laser ablation requires prior endometrial sampling
C perforation occurs in 5% of cases
D resection of submucous fibroids is possible
E hyponatraemia is a recognized side effect

6.35 In applied pharmacology of the renal tract

A PGs have been shown to decrease spontaneous detrusor contractions
B phenoxybenzamine and prazosin are used to facilitate bladder emptying when there is bladder neck outlet obstruction
C tachyphylaxis limits the long-term use of phenylpropanolamine in women with stress incontinence
D oxybutynin will facilitate bladder storage of urine and acts as a local anaesthetic on the bladder
E intranasal desmopressin is useful in the management of nocturia in the hypertensive patient

6.36 Regarding pelvic inflammatory disease

A postpartum infection is the commonest aetiological factor
B laparoscopy should be deferred in suspected PID due to the risk of dissemination of infection
C all suspected cases should have a vaginal swab for bacteriological analysis
D chronic PID may present with non-specific symptoms and anaemia
E hysterectomy with ovarian conservation may be performed in a young woman with symptoms not relieved by prolonged antibiotic therapy

6.37 Pelvic venous congestion

A common in menopausal women
B characterized by a dull aching pain with acute exacerbations
C hysterectomy results in almost universal cure
D progestogens have long-term benefit
E ergot alkaloids have short-term effects

• 6.38 In determining the exact diagnosis of urinary incontinence

A it is known that vaginal delivery is the commonest cause of urethral sphincter incompetence
B voiding greater than 10/day is defined as frequency
C at least 60% of patients with urethral sphincter incompetence have significant anterior vaginal wall descent
D a simple neurological examination should be performed to screen all such patients
E treatments by placebo drugs have been shown to produce improvement rates of 50% in women with detrusor instability

• 6.39 Gestational trophoblastic disease

A a partial mole may coexist with a fetus *in utero*
B invasive mole penetrates the myometrium and has identifiable chorionic villi
C commonly comprises cells with 46XX chromosomes of paternal origin
D has a greater than 20-fold increase in incidence in mothers over 45 years old
E after evacuation of a hydatidiform mole the patient is monitored using urinary beta-hCG assays

6.40　Polycystic ovary syndrome

A　anovulation can be treated with clomiphene
B　the risk of endometrial cancer is decreased
C　Metrodin is contraindicated for ovulation induction
D　hyperthyroidism should be excluded
E　cyproterone acetate is used to treat hirsutism

6.41　In HIV infection in women

A　the average interval between viral infection and the onset of AIDS is 8 years
B　menstrual abnormalities are more common in intravenous drug abusers than in matched controls
C　vertical transmission in pregnancy in the Western world is of the order of 20%
D　the condom is the contraceptive of choice
E　a low CD4 count is associated with an increased risk of other serious infections

6.42　Carcinoma of the vulva

A　causes over 1000 deaths per annum in England and Wales
B　is related to HPV infection in a proportion of cases
C　melanomata comprise about 10% of vulval cancers
D　has a peak incidence in the fifth and sixth decades of life
E　VIN is a premalignant condition and is due to cell changes occurring in areas of lichen sclerosus

6.43　Fibroids can result in

A　menorrhagia in all cases
B　polycythemia
C　constipation
D　acute urinary retention
E　infertility due to impaired implantation

6.44 Mifepristone

A a 19 keto-steroid, is the first antiprogestogen to become available for routine clinical use in the UK
B acts as a competitive receptor antagonist with a three- to five-fold greater receptor affinity than progesterone
C may also affect glucocorticoid receptor binding
D use is contraindicated in women greater than 35 years of age or women who smoke greater than 10 cigarettes per day
E may be used to treat malignant disease of the breast and meninges

6.45 Male subfertility

A surgery to correct a blocked vas deferens after tuberculosis is more successful than vasectomy reversal
B the first sample in a split ejaculate has a relatively low concentration of spermatozoa
C impotence is the common presenting symptom in hyperprolactinaemia
D treatment of antisperm antibodies with high-dose steroids may result in pregnancy but there is a significant incidence of complications, notably femoral head necrosis
E IVF for oligospermia may result in pregnancy when a prepared semen sample contains as few as 50 000 spermatozoa per ml

6.46 The following drugs can result in hyperprolactinaemia

A methyldopa
B atenolol
C metoclopramide
D cimetidine
E diazepam

6.47 Vaginal hysterectomy

A should not be performed if the uterus is greater than 14 weeks in size
B is more likely to result in ureteric injury than during abdominal hysterectomy
C has a mortality rate of 1:10 000 patients
D should ideally be preceded by a D&C to exclude an endometrial malignancy
E is normally only possible in a multiparous woman with good access and at least type I uterine descent

6.48 Ovarian tumours

A endometrioid tumours arise in epithelial cells
B borderline tumours are of germ cell origin
C choriocarcinoma of ovarian germ cell origin responds readily to methotrexate
D dermoid cysts are more common in elderly women
E Brenner tumours arise in epithelial cells of Wolffian origin

6.49 The following can result in chronic pelvic pain

A uterovaginal prolapse
B residual ovary syndrome
C retroverted uterus
D Crohn's disease
E PCOS

6.50 Menorrhagia

A is defined as menstrual blood loss in excess of 100 ml per period
B has no underlying organic pathology or abnormality of the hypothalamic–pituitary–ovarian–uterine axis in the majority of cases
C is primarily due to components of the endometrial fibrinolytic system and/or prostaglandins
D treated by mefenamic acid is cheaper and associated with fewer side effects than if treated with danazol
E treated with GnRH analogues may result in hypo-oestrogenism which can be diminished by the concomitant administration of synthetic ovarian steroids

6.51 Tumours which commonly arise in the vagina include

A dermoid cysts
B sarcoma botrioydes
C Gartner's duct adenoma
D clear cell adenocarcinoma
E Brenner tumour

6.52 The following are symptoms of premenstrual syndrome

A breast tenderness
B menorrhagia
C weight loss
D change in libido
E acne

6.53 In childhood

A ovarian malignancy is the commonest gynaecological neoplasm
B an asymptomatic mass is the commonest presentation of gynaecological malignancy
C in girls less than 15 years old, survival after clear cell adenocarcinoma of the vagina is comparable to survival after squamous cell carcinoma of the cervix
D radiation therapy for gynaecological malignancy is associated with an increased incidence of premature menopause
E ovarian dysgerminoma is bilateral in 30% of cases

6.54 In determining the level of a substance in the body

A immunoassays measure the equilibrium between the hormone to be measured and an antibody, with a tracer attached to either
B agglutination assays are more sensitive than immunoassays
C a deficiency of the thyroid hormones leads to anovulation and raised gonadotrophin levels
D assaying the products of the adrenal zona fasciculata will establish cortisol levels
E circulating AFP levels in a normal pregnant woman continue to rise until 36 weeks

6.55 PCOS can be associated with

A FSH:LH ratio of 3:1
B raised testosterone
C lowered oestrone
D raised prolactin
E raised androstenedione

6.56   Laparoscopic hysterectomy

A is an alternative to abdominal and vaginal hysterectomy

B patients require one-third of the average postoperative opiate analgesia required by a patient who has undergone an abdominal hysterectomy

C is associated with a reduction in the length of hospitalization and postoperative recovery

D should not be performed if there is malignant pathology

E is associated with less blood loss than in conventional surgery

6.57   In the management of benign uterine tumours

A an LHRH analogue may be useful in decreasing the size of a fibroid prior to surgery

B localized pain and tenderness in the gravid uterus may be due to red degeneration of a fibroid

C it is known that indigenous Nigerian women have a reduced incidence of uterine fibroids

D cigarette smokers have an increased incidence of fibroids

E HRT administration to postmenopausal women with fibroids is contraindicated

6.58   A laser

A can produce visible and invisible beams of light

B is an acronym for light acceleration by the stimulated emission of radiation

C when used with CO_2 is focused using an articulated arm with a mirror at each joint

D must be operated within strictly defined regulations and, in particular, maximum permitted exposure (MPE) levels must be observed

E does not cause thermal damage to surrounding tissue

6.59   In recurrent gynaecological malignancy

A the commonest indication for pelvic exenterative surgery is ovarian malignancy

B metastatic bone disease is uncommon in cervical cancer

C further radical surgery should not be carried out on psychotic patients

D urinary diversion using a jejunal conduit has been abandoned because of the significant electrolyte imbalances associated with its use

E the construction of a neovagina is essential in the psychosexual rehabilitation of some patients after vaginal exenterative surgery

6.60 **In gestational trophoblastic disease**

    A hydropic degeneration and placental site reaction inevitably proceed to malignancy

    B placental site trophoblastic tumour characteristically has very high levels of beta-hCG

    C choriocarcinoma may be excluded by a normal serum beta-hCG level

    D the three drugs with the greatest activity against such malignant tumours are methotrexate, actinomycin-D and etoposide

    E the incidence is 1–2/1000 live births and increases with decreasing maternal age

ANSWERS TO PAPER ONE

The correct answers appear in bold
References refer to page numbers in *Key Topics in Obstetrics and Gynaecology* and references on p. 141 of this book

1.1 **A B D** p.146
    C more common in multiparity
    E associated with ARM or following SROM

1.2 **A** p.276; see also [1] p.169 and [2] p.122
    B T4, T3 and TBG all rise, with TBG rise being due to increased hepatic synthesis in the presence of increased oestrogens
    C it lies between the first and second pharyngeal pouches
    D the placenta does produce thyroid-like stimulating substances but they do not act upon the thyroid itself
    E thyroid hormones maintain phospholipid synthesis and do not initiate type II pneumocyte activity

1.3 **A C** p.261
    B the baby should be observed for drowsiness
    D mothers over age 30 form a high-risk group
    E the incidence varies up to around 24%

1.4 **C** p.151
    A TENS electrodes are placed over T10–L1 and S2–S4
    B Entonox is 50:50 oxygen and nitrous oxide
    D pethidine reduces scores by only 20%
    E pethidine reduces gastric emptying

1.5 **C E** p.272; see also [3] p.4
    A maternal death is defined as death of a woman during pregnancy or before the 42nd postpartum day
    B fortuitous deaths are maternal deaths from causes not related to or influenced by the pregnancy
    D the Report on Confidential Enquiries into Maternal Deaths began in 1952, whilst NCEPOD only began in 1992

1.6 **B E** p.193
    A polyglycolic acid (Dexon) has been shown to be superior in terms of short-term pain
    C subcuticular skin suturing minimises early discomfort; there is no evidence of any improvement in late discomfort
    D in general a neat incision is preferable to a ragged tear; as it is easier to repair, complications should be reduced

1.7 C D E p.157
    A APH is associated with a blood loss in excess of 15 ml
    B frequency of placenta praevia is 0.4–0.8%

1.8 B D E See [4] p.263
    A it is 3 cm long
    C it is more than halved

1.9 E p.256
    A mentoanterior position is likely to result in spontaneous vaginal delivery
    B experienced operators may effect rotation to the occipitoanterior position
    C the occiput is the denominator in normal labour
    D deep transverse arrest may be overcome with intravenous Syntocinon

1.10 A C D p.160
    B fetal growth can be calculated but is not part of the BPP
    E umbilical cord Doppler is not used for the BPP

1.11 A B E See [6] p.99
    C 4–6% of all newborn Down's syndrome babies are due to a translocation trisomy
    D the IQ is within the normal range, as are the emotions and the psychological behaviour of Turner's syndrome people

1.12 A B C D E p.185

1.13 B C p.162
    A occurs in only 16% of cases at 32 weeks
    D at term 4% of pregnancies are breech
    E bitrochanteric diameter is 9.25 cm with the biparietal diameter being 9.5 cm

1.14 C D E p.268; see also [2] p.641
    A they have a greater than 30% chance
    B in general, azathioprine and cyclosporin A are not thought to be teratogenic, and should be continued throughout the pregnancy to protect the transplant

1.15 D p.274
    A the rhesus antigen is located on chromosome 1
    B the D gene is the most clinically relevant
    C cordocentesis has an abortion rate of the order of 2%; amniocentesis is the standard investigation
    E irradiation of donor blood for intrauterine transfusion is standard practice in some centres

1.16 A C D E p.174
> B bone formation is dependent on vitamin D and phosphorus

1.17 C E p.154; and see also [2] p.993 and [7] p.338
> A viscerocranium, not somatocranium
> B the posterior fontanelle is triangular
> D the BPD at term is 9.5 cm

1.18 A E p.224
> B older mothers are more likely to have multiple pregnancy
> C beta-adrenergics may be recommended in triplet and quad pregnancy
> D there is no increase in antepartum haemorrhage in multiple pregnancy

1.19 A D E p.188
> B trigone is mesodermal in origin
> C ureters will arise from the metanephros

1.20 A D E p.171
> B 7% mortality
> C provided therapeutic maternal digoxin levels are maintained, there is no risk of digoxin toxicity to the fetus

1.21 C D p.221
> A the Dublin trial shows no benefit of continuous monitoring by CTG over intermittent fetal heart auscultation
> B the correlation between abnormal CTG and a hypoxic fetal blood sample is low (<53%)
> E continuous monitoring, preferably by internal tocography is generally recommended in high-risk labour; fetal blood samples are taken as indicated

1.22 A B D E p.191
> C increased risk of abruption but not placenta praevia

1.23 A C p.179
> B facilitated diffusion, not active transport
> D HbA_{1C} needs to be greater than 10%
> E a WHO GTT involves giving 75 g of oral glucose

1.24 A E p.165
> B classical section may be performed via a Pfannenstiel incision, the uterine incision determines the nature of the operation
> C a trial of labour may be allowed if pelvimetry and fetal weight are compatible with possible vaginal delivery
> D the classical procedure cannot be justified on grounds of speed; it is used when the lower segment has not formed

1.25 A C D E p.197
B the uterus should be contracting

1.26 A B C D p.200; see also [9] p.5 and [10] Part 1, p.2
E there are no reported home confinement maternal deaths

1.27 A E p.210
B ophthalmia neonatorum is caused by direct transmission during parturition
C there is an effective screening and immunization programme for congenital rubella; cytomegalovirus is the commonest pathogen
D this is suggestive of listeriosis

1.28 A B D E p.197
C symphysiotomy is almost never performed in the UK but is often performed in developing countries

1.29 B C p.205
A cell-mediated immunity, not humoral immunity
D the placenta lacks detectable expression of class II MHC (HLA transplantation) antigens
E the IgG autoantibodies may cross the placenta and involve the fetus

1.30 A B p.229
C the biparietal diameter reaches the introitus at crowning
D oxytocic agents are given with delivery of the anterior shoulder
E the incidence of retained placenta is reduced with active management

1.31 A B C D E p.203

1.32 B C E p.226
A reflex irritability, not reflex grasping
D greater than 340 μmol/l, not greater than 300 μmol/l

1.33 A B C p.144
D in the absence of a predisposing cause, hypotonic activity is largely confined to primigravidae
E nerve supply to the myometrium is sparse; stimulation is largely biochemical and hormonal

1.34 C D p.214
A fetal heart sounds can often be difficult to pick up
B fetal movements can stop spasmodically throughout pregnancy
E fetal bladder can be empty

1.35 B C D p.231
    A the average weight gain is 12.5 kg
    E there is an increase, not a decrease in the blood volume

1.36 A C D E p.148
    B the most efficiently absorbed dietary iron is in animal haemoglobin and myoglobin

1.37 A C D E p.217
    B larger babies are more common in subsequent pregnancies

1.38 B p.242
    A 5–10% are affected
    C the diagnosis is generally made greater than 20 weeks, but rarely can be made less than 20 weeks
    D proteinuria should be greater than 300 mg/24 h
    E greater than 2 kg/week weight gain is significant

1.39 C E p.168
    A cancer complicates about 1 in 1000 pregnancies
    B dilation of the cervix is said to cause dissemination of malignant cells
    D there is no change in survival stage for stage

1.40 A B C E p.235
    D Potter's syndrome is associated with oligohydramnios

1.41 B C D p.259
    A prolonged pregnancy is not synonymous with postmaturity
    E 15% when the dates are uncertain

1.42 D p.176
    A there is no significant change
    B the main increases are in factors II, VII, VIII and X
    C there is no detectable plasminogen activity
    E these changes result in increased blood flow

1.43 A C E p.237
    B postmaturity does not result in a PPH
    D PPH is associated with multiparity

1.44 A B C E p.265
    D 15%

1.45 A C p.263
    B these are late signs of abscess formation and septicaemia
    D treatment is promptly instituted with broad-spectrum antibiotics
    E an abscess is treated by incision and drainage

1.46 **B C D E** p.245

    A obesity does not result in premature labour

1.47 **A** p.266

    B oxytocin is manufactured in the hypothalamus

    C 800–1200 ml per day

    D oxytocin is an octapeptide

    E dopamine is inhibitory to prolactin

1.48 **A B C E** p.176

    D heparin does not cross the placenta

1.49 **A B D** p.248

    C coital activity is not associated with PROM

    E amniotic fluid has a pH greater than 7.1 with nitrazine sticks going black

1.50 **C D** p.141

    A T10 to L1

    B the maternal mortality is greater than 10%

    E the appendix rises with gestation

1.51 **A B C** p.185

    D not a recognized association

    E not a recognized association

1.52 **A C** p.250

    B synthesized in yolk sac, fetal liver and by 17 weeks in fetal CSF

    D open neural tube defects result in raised AFP

    E trisomy 21 results in a lowered AFP

1.53 **A B D E** See [13] p.159

    C oxytocin also increases the duration

1.54 **A C D E** p.263

    B in the absence of associated symptoms it is preferable to await results of bacteriological investigation

1.55 **A B D** p.250

    C large choroid plexus cysts are associated with chromosomal problems

    E open spina bifida has a worse prognosis

1.56 **A B C E** See [13] p.213

    D epidural anaesthesia is safe

1.57 **E** p.210
- A the risk is estimated at 22–51%
- B only if persistently elevated
- C there appears to be no adverse effect related to pregnancy
- D the main risks are related to prematurity and growth retardation

1.58 **A B D** p.250
- C only usually offered in those women who have already had a Down's child
- E this has not been a reported side effect

1.59 **A B C D E** See [13] pp.13–31 and [16] p.247

1.60 **A C D** p.176
- B warfarin should be stopped near to delivery as its anticoagulant effect is not easily reversible
- E heparin may only be administered by injection

ANSWERS TO PAPER TWO

The correct answers appear in bold
References refer to page numbers in *Key Topics in Obstetrics and Gynaecology* and references on p. 141 of this book

2.1 **A B C E** p.146
      D mortality rate is over 80%

2.2 **A D** See [2] p.121
      B the Regional Obstetric Assessor is responsible for compiling the Report
      C the District Coroner's Report is not included in the Regional Obstetric Assessor's Report
      E strict confidentiality is maintained at all stages of the Confidential Enquiries, the identity of the patient is erased from all forms so that the opinion of the Assessors cannot be traced back to an identified individual and after the completion of each Triennial Report all MCW97 Enquiry Forms are destroyed

2.3 **A B C D E** p.240

2.4 **A B C D** p.151
      E Mendelson's syndrome occurs with GA

2.5 **B E** See [6] pp.147, 315, 425, 441 and 461
      A DNA not RNA
      C Southern blot analysis
      D Duchenne's muscular dystrophy affects males, not females

2.6 **C D** p.183
      A Montgomery's tubercles on the nipple become increasingly prominent during pregnancy
      B nausea and vomiting may occur at any time
      E the beta subunit of hCG is specific

2.7 **A B D E** p.157
      C more common in multiparity

2.8 **A C E** p. 154; see also [8] p. 282
      B the crista dividens preferentially diverts blood from the IVC through the foramen ovale into the left atrium
      D the single umbilical vein carrying oxygenated blood leaves the placenta, whilst the two umbilical arteries return deoxygenated blood to the placenta

2.9 B C D E p.185

A low-dose aspirin is recommended under these circumstances

2.10 A C D E p.160

B chronic hypoxia results in oligohydramnios and extrinsic growth failure

2.11 B C p.179; see also [2] p.595

A there is a 7% chance
D she should be seen yearly by an ophthalmologist
E there is a 14.4% prevalence of pre-eclampsia in diabetics

2.12 A B C p.261

D electroconvulsive therapy is a standard form of treatment
E it is commoner in mothers over age 30

2.13 A C D E p.162

B breech is more common if the legs are extended

2.14 A B C p.195

D isoimmunization can occur during a normal vaginal delivery
E IgM cannot cross the placenta, rather IgG does in this case

2.15 A B p.165

C the ureters are at risk during suturing of a lateral extension of a transverse incision
D as most surgeons are more familiar with the lower segment approach little is to be gained on grounds of speed
E although many surgeons practice this manoeuvre it is not essential

2.16 A D E p.174

B Afro-Caribbean women commonly have a high angle of inclination of their pelvis and this can be associated with a high head at term
C engagement should occur after 39 weeks

2.17 B C E p.207

A prostaglandins prime the uterus for oxytocin action as a secondary event
D there is an increase in the compliance of the cervix

2.18 D p.229

A the classic definition is of progressive dilatation
B retraction is a normal occurrence
C average time is 30 min
E placental blood is dark red

2.19 A B C E p.188

D paramesonephric ducts are lateral to the mesonephric ducts

2.20 **A B** pp.227 and 245
   C the frequency in term infants is 0.01%
   D necrotising pneumonitis does not occur
   E the CXR has a 'ground glass' appearance

2.21 **A D** p.224
   B there is a five-fold increase
   C prematurity is the main aetiological factor
   E fetal maturity is the main prognostic factor

2.22 **A B D E** p.192
   C club foot is not increased

2.23 **A C D** p.232
   B the WHO definition of anaemia in pregnancy is less than 11.0 g/dl
   E the fourth Korotkoff sound should be used

2.24 **B C D** p.274
   A inheritance is by simple Mendelian principles
   E anti-D is administered to at-risk women providing passive immunization

2.25 **A B D** p.197
   C perineal damage is three-fold more in forceps deliveries than ventouse
   E cephalohaematomas usually occupy the parietal bones

2.26 **A** p.242
   B the aim is to stabilize the maternal condition before delivery
   C magnesium sulphate is advocated by some
   D delivery should be by Caesarean section under general anaesthesia
   E eclamptics may be asymptomatic

2.27 **C** p.148
   A crises occur more frequently
   B SC disease is a mild form of sickle cell anaemia but crises occur in pregnancy
   D alpha-thalassaemia major is incompatible with life
   E thalassaemias are due to impaired globin synthesis

2.28 **A B C D E** p.274; see also [2] pp.623 and 991

2.29 **B C E** See [13] p.183
   A centimetres, not inches
   D they are more common after vacuum extraction

2.30 D p.144
A hypotonic activity is more common
B the reverse is true
C this is contraindicated
E stress is related to hypotonicity

2.31 A B D p.214
C 90% of patients will deliver within 3 weeks
E karyotype parents only if fetus is abnormal

2.32 A C p.203
B polyhydramnios is present and has a pool depth of at least 8 cm
D diaphragmatic hernias are associated with hydrops but not always
E cordocentesis is only indicated if an infective or chromosomal cause is suspected

2.33 A D E p.183
B urinary frequency occurs from about 8 weeks
C amenorrhoea occurs 14 days postfertilization

2.34 A B C E p.217
D USS is the best way of detecting IUGR

2.35 C D See [2] p.383 and [14] Ch. 22, 24, 27
A maternal vascular response
B 2–8 cm is the normal range
E symptomatic polyhydramnios

2.36 A B p.193
C anal and/or rectal mucosal damage constitutes a third-degree tear
D the posterior fourchette is the site of every episiotomy incision
E subcuticular suturing with polyglycolic acid is superior in this respect

2.37 A B C E p.237
D associated with polyhydramnios

2.38 C p.154; see also [12] p.2 and [15] p.32
A posterior border of the symphysis pubis
B they should be at least 11.5 cm
D the nerve lies medial to the artery
E the angle of inclination should be 135°

2.39 A B D E p.210
C it may be passive immunity; infection is likely if it persists beyond 9 months

2.40 A C D p.245
   B fetal distress is also a contraindication
   E vertex presentations are allowed to be delivered vaginally

2.41 A B D E p.276; see also [2] p.453
   C medical treatment with carbimazole is the treatment of choice

2.42 C D p.168
   A the prognosis is worse
   B pregnancy has occurred after chemotherapy for Hodgkin's disease
   E careful supervision is necessary but pregnancy may be allowed

2.43 A C D E p.248
   B corticosteroids should always be administered before 34 weeks

2.44 B C D E See [13] p.33
   A reduction in osmotic pressure (hypoproteinaemia), not hepatic failure

2.45 B E p.221
   A a fetal scalp electrode for continuous internal monitoring is applied
      when possible
   C this level warrants close observation but not delivery
   D complicated baseline tachycardia is the most ominous pattern

2.46 A B C E p.250
   D Down's syndrome is associated with a lowered AFP

2.47 A B C D E See [13] p.135

2.48 A p.240
   B the aim of counselling should be a positive effect
   C control of blood sugar should begin before conception to reduce the
      incidence of congenital anomalies
   D the primary consideration is the mother's drug requirements; risks
      should be quantified where possible
   E physiological changes in pregnancy may lead to cardiac failure

2.49 B E p.250
   A cystic hygroma is not always associated with Turner's syndrome but it
      does raise a suspicion of Turner's and also of trisomy 21
   C diaphragmatic hernia is recurrent
   D gastroschisis is not associated with chromosomal abnormalities

2.50 A B C D E See [13] p.87

2.51 A D p.148
  B fetal iron requirements are maximal at 32 weeks gestation
  C women have a precarious iron balance due to continued menstrual loss; therefore iron deficiency is less likely if oligomenorrhoeic women become pregnant
  E a reduction in serum ferritin is a sensitive indicator of deficient iron stores and indicates those at risk of developing iron deficiency anaemia

2.52 B C D E p.250
  A can be performed transcervically

2.53 D p.256
  A breech extraction is unsafe in a singleton delivery
  B the malpresentation usually corrects and leads to a vaginal delivery
  C vaginal delivery is only possible in a face in a mentoanterior position
  E they are associated with android, anthropoid and platypelloid pelvises

2.54 B C D E p.176
  A is always secondary to an external predisposing cause

2.55 A C D p.157
  B associated with a raised AFP
  E occurs in association with polyhydramnios

2.56 A D E p.253
  B there should be less than 1% losses
  C it must be performed under USS guidance

2.57 A B C E p.185
  D naloxone reverses opiate-induced neonatal respiratory depression

2.58 A C D p.235
  B oligohydramnios is associated with a raised AFP
  E multiple pregnancy is associated with polyhydramnios

2.59 D E p.191
  A the incidence is 1:40
  B carbamazepine is the drug of choice
  C folate deficiency

2.60 A B C E p.148
  D individuals with beta-thalassaemia major may survive with repeated blood transfusions

ANSWERS TO PAPER THREE

The correct answers appear in bold

References refer to page numbers in *Key Topics in Obstetrics and Gynaecology* and references on p. 141 of this book

3.1 **A B C D E** p.146

3.2 **A E** p.155
- B increase in pCO_2 with delivery
- C medial umbilical ligaments, not the lateral
- D decrease in IVC blood pressure

3.3 **A** p.256
- B common compound presentations such as a hand beside the head usually correct spontaneously
- C an anthropoid pelvis is associated with malposition
- D no
- E this is dangerous; cord prolapse is excluded and arrangements made for Caesarean section unless the presentation is breech

3.4 **A C E** p.151; see also [13] p.183
- B minimized by left lateral tilt
- D previous Caesarean section is not a contraindication

3.5 **B D E** p.181; see [2] p.600
- A pregnancy may be continued up to 40 completed weeks safely
- C the blood glucose ideally should remain between 4 and 6 mmol/l

3.6 **A B E** p.263
- C not an indication *per se*
- D a slightly unlikely situation, i.e. membranes should be ruptured before four vaginal examinations are necessary but the risk of sepsis is low

3.7 **A B C** p.157
- D abruption is classically painful
- E bleeding can occur in approximately 10% of pregnancies

3.8 **A D** p.207
- B free calcium ions, not bound ones
- C 0.2% hypertonus risk
- E it is prostaglandin synthetase inhibitors, e.g. indomethacin, that carry a risk of premature closure of the ductus and not prostaglandins themselves

3.9   B C D E p.144

    A the unit of measurement is kPa/15 min

3.10   C p.160

    A the BPP is made up of five components

    B not if oligohydramnios is present

    D amniotic fluid volume is important in chronic hypoxia

    E Doppler flow recordings do not contribute to the BPP

3.11   C D E p.232

    A the anteroposterior diameter increases

    B the respiratory rate remains approximately constant

3.12   C D E p.256

    A this is not an indication for induction

    B if labour is progressing at an acceptable rate there is no need for
       augmentation

3.13   A D p.162

    B fetal weight should be below 3500 g but this is not mandatory

    C Syntocinon augmentation is only contraindicated in the second stage

    E a flat sacrum is not ideal for a vaginal breech delivery

3.14   A C p.244

    B haemolysis, not haematemesis

    D low-dose aspirin is 60–75 mg/day

    E there is no definite cause yet known in pre-eclampsia

3.15   A C E p.210

    B immune mothers may suffer re-infection

    D up to 90% of affected babies show no sign of congenital anomaly at
       birth

3.16   A C D E p.174

    B a well-applied cervix is associated with well-progressing labour

3.17   A C D p.242; see also [2] p.519 and [12] p.1035

    B urate and creatinine assess renal function

    E macrocytic, not microcytic

3.18   A B p.274

    C the antibody is measured by direct assay

    D inheritance is by Mendelian principles, the figure is 100%

    E routine antibody estimation is performed at regular intervals as there is a
       risk of silent sensitization

3.19 A B C E p.188

D urethra develops from the mesonephric ducts and the urogenital sinus

3.20 C D E p.243; see also [2] p.528

A in general, hypertension does not need treatment until it reaches greater than 170/110 mmHg

B after IV administration there is a significant delay of 20–30 min before its onset of action

3.21 A B p.210

C this has been shown to be of no clinical value

D Caesarean section is not indicated after the membranes have been ruptured for 4 hours as fetal infection is likely to have already occurred

E primary genital herpes gives rise to serious neonatal infection in 50% of cases

3.22 A B D E p.191

C CTGs can become unreactive if anticonvulsant therapy is present

3.23 C D E See [13] p.183

A there is no true descent

B Caesarean section should be performed

3.24 D p.168

A Caesarean Wertheim's hysterectomy is frequently performed

B the prognosis is unaltered stage for stage

C there are around 40 reported cases

E the radiation field is remote from the fetus and pregnancy may continue if the fetus is adequately protected

3.25 A B C D E p.197

3.26 B C D E p.268

A the GFR is 60% greater than normal at 16 weeks gestation

3.27 D E p.221

A cardiotocography has a high false-positive rate (there is an error in the first edition of *Key Topics* on this point)

B this is a high-risk labour; continuous monitoring is recommended

C this method is invasive and intrusive

3.28 B C D E p.203

A hydrops fetalis may cause pre-eclampsia but not vice versa

3.29 **B C E** See [13] p.13
  A multiples of the median
  D chorionic villus biopsy performed under 10 weeks gestation may result in the oromandibular limb hypoplasia syndrome

3.30 **A B E** p.274
  C the appearances are of a large-for-dates and oedematous fetus
  D Liley charts are for plotting amniotic fluid bilirubin levels

3.31 **A D E** p.214
  B LSCS may be necessary in exceptional cases, e.g. major placenta praevia
  C ARM is performed in established labour

3.32 **B C** See [13] p.135
  A 70% chance of recurring
  D such an infection is significant and warrants treatment
  E bacteria can cross intact membranes

3.33 **A** p.224
  B the glomerular filtration rate is increased
  C although carrying a high mortality, locked twins are rare
  D the aim of bed rest in triplet pregnancy is to reduce the incidence of premature labour
  E malpresentation of the first twin is an indication for elective Caesarean section (breech presentation may be an exception)

3.34 **A E** p.217
  B crown–rump length is accurate to within 3 days
  C best estimate of fetal weight is obtained by the abdominal circumference
  D symmetrical IUGR is associated with intrinsic cause such as trisomy 21

3.35 **A B C** p.250
  D there is a single centrally placed ventricle
  E gastroschisis has a better prognosis than omphalocele

3.36 **A** p.183
  B the reverse is usually the case
  C this usually occurs from 12 weeks
  D Hegar's sign is unnecessarily traumatic
  E the beta subunit of hCG is specific

3.37 **A B C E** p.237
  D internal iliac ligation is performed

3.38 p.250
   A amniocentesis is safer than chorionic villus biopsy
   B there is a loss rate of around 4%
   C it should be performed at greater than 10/40 gestation
   D mosaicism may occur
   E the transabdominal approach should be used

3.39 **B D** p.261
   A the commonest complaint is of a persistent lowering of mood
   C this is a common aetiological factor, not a symptom
   E prompt treatment with antidepressants may be beneficial

3.40 **B C E** p.237
   A secondary PPH has a prevalence of 0.5–1.5%
   D occurs during the second week after delivery

3.41 **A B** p.237
   C Jehovah's Witnesses will refuse a blood transfusion
   D ligation of the internal iliac artery
   E it is not a secondary PPH at 10 weeks

3.42 **A** p.176
   B this occurs in placental vessels
   C bed rest predisposes to venous stasis
   D a suspected pulmonary embolus should be promptly treated with
     intravenous heparin
   E protamine sulphate is a heparin antagonist; the treatment is vitamin K

3.43 **A B C D** p.245
   E regular uterine contractions before 37 completed weeks

3.44 **B C E** p.197
   A Wrigley's forceps have a fixed pivot lock
   D one-fifth palpable per abdomen is acceptable for a vaginal delivery

3.45 **B D E** p.168
   A management is by a multidisciplinary approach, including obstetrician,
     surgeon, medical oncologist and radiotherapist where appropriate and
     should take place in a specialist centre
   C gonadotrophins have a TSH-like effect

3.46 **A C D** p.248
   B LSCS indicated for breech estimated to weigh 800–1500 g
   E PROM often results with no other symptom

3.47 **D E** p.183
A Montgomery's tubercles are only a sign and do not make the diagnosis
B the beta subunit of hCG
C Hegar's sign detection is traumatic and unnecessary

3.48 **A C D E** p.274
B amniocentesis is less accurate but has a lower complication rate

3.49 **B C** p.250
A posterior valves can rarely occur in the female fetus
D oligohydramnios has many other causes
E polyhydramnios does not occur in lower bowel blockage such as an imperforate anus

3.50 **A B C D E** p.193

3.51 **A E** p.185
B methotrexate is a cytotoxic drug and is absolutely contraindicated
C papaveretum is not recommended as it contains the teratogen noscapine
D carbamazepine has fewer adverse effects

3.52 **A B D E** p.250
C CVS is used primarily as first choice in metabolic disorders

3.53 **E** p.207
A greater than 95% go into established labour
B meta-analysis has shown vaginal prostaglandins to be safe in the presence of ruptured membranes
C there is no significant difference in the cord gases in such cases
D the failure rate is 2–5%

3.54 **A** p.144
B hypertonic uterine activity has this effect
C reversal occurs at about 5 min
D commonly iatrogenic, rarely idiopathic
E calculation of intrauterine pressure requires a normal baseline uterine muscle tone

3.55 **A C D E** p.250
B a high hCG is associated with Down's syndrome

3.56 **B D E** p.248
A the pH is 7.1
C coital activity is not linked with preterm rupture of the membranes

3.57 **C D E** p.148
A vitamin B12 stores are usually adequate
B folate deficiency is associated with lower social classes

3.58 A C E p.235
    B diabetes mellitus is associated with polyhydramnios
    D trisomy 21 does not result in oligohydramnios

3.59 A B D p.162
    C epidural anaesthesia is often advisable for a vaginal breech delivery
    E Syntocinon should only be given in first stage

3.60 B C D p.245
    A only more common in multigravidae if previous history
    E can result in oligohydramnios

ANSWERS TO PAPER FOUR

The correct answers appear in bold

References refer to page numbers in *Key Topics in Obstetrics and Gynaecology* and references on p. 141 of this book

4.1 B C E p.1
  A 72% of hysterectomies are abdominal
  D vault prolapse occurs in less than 2%

4.2 A B D E See [12] p.623
  C urinary incontinence is defined as an involuntary loss of urine which is objectively demonstrable and a social or hygienic problem

4.3 A E p.6
  B the commonest reason for outflow obstruction is anatomical, with normal female hormone levels
  C it is unwise to inform the patient if genotypically male or to attempt to change the sex of rearing
  D successful treatment with dilators requires a highly motivated patient

4.4 A B p.3
  C incidence between 30 and 40%
  D threatened abortion must have a viable pregnancy
  E risk of abortion after positive ultrasound is 5%

4.5 D E See [12] p.637
  A detrusor instability is not usually clearly defined
  B any such surgery may increase the incidence of detrusor instability
  C coital incontinence is found

4.6 B p.117
  A there was one reported case of congenital syphilis in 1983
  C chlamydial organisms contain both DNA and RNA
  D chlamydiae are often found in association with gonorrhoea
  E beta-lactamase strains of gonorrhoea are penicillin resistant

4.7 A B D p.9
  C treatment of an abscess is by marsupialization
  E most superficial infections are treated in the community by antibiotics

4.8 B C p.154; see also [12] p.23
  A the pudendal nerve innervates the external anal sphincter
  D there is no known true internal urethral sphincter
  E it is most at risk as it crosses the bifurcation of the common iliac artery

4.9   p.138

    A the presence of HPV is associated with coexistent cellular atypia
    B diagnosis is by biopsy; examination is unreliable
    C hypertrophic dystrophy is associated with elongation of rete ridges
    D steroid creams are indicated for severe inflammatory changes
    E skinning vulvectomy has a high recurrence rate (>50%)

4.10 **B C D E** p.17

    A spasm of the pubococcygeus is a cause of vaginismus not dyspareunia

4.11 **D** See [1] pp.1083 and 1328

    A the ureters are 30–35 cm long
    B the ureter is crossed by the ovarian vessels in its abdominal course
    C there is no intimal layer
    E T11–L2 innervation

4.12 **C D E** p.59

    A there is a male factor in over 1 in 3 couples seeking treatment for
       subfertility
    B psychosexual problems in the male rarely present to infertility clinics

4.13 **A B C E** p.19

    D combined oral contraceptive pill protects against ectopic pregnancy

4.14 **C D E** See [1] p.1377 and [12] p.313

    A androgens are secreted from the two inner zones, the zona fasciculata
       and the zona reticularis
    B 25% comes from the adrenals, 25% from the ovaries and 50% from
       extraglandular sources

4.15 **B C D** p.22

    A the most widely held theory is of direct implantation of endometrial
       cells after retrograde menstruation
    E recent studies do not confirm the role of prostaglandins with relation to
       ovum release and tubal motility

4.16 **A D E** p.29

    B sarcomatous change occurs in 0.2%
    C only 30% of fibroids are submucous and result in menorrhagia

4.17 **A B C** See [12] p.313

    D cyproterone acetate is an antiandrogenic progestogen; it is however
       useful in the treatment of the hirsute patient
    E spironolactone can interfere with sexual differentiation of a male fetus;
       thus, it must be used in conjunction with a contraceptive during
       hirsutism treatment if the patient is at risk of becoming pregnant

4.18 B C D E p.78

    A the oral contraceptive pill exerts a protective effect

4.19 B C p.32

    A commonest UK cause is surgical misadventure

    D direct visualization and contrast radiography are better

    E congenital defects are rare

4.20 B C p.44

    A HRT is not contraceptive in any premenopausal woman

    D opposed HRT protects against endometrial hyperplasia

    E there is no guarantee of complete endometrial resection/ablation with such techniques and there is therefore a risk of endometrial hyperplasia or frank malignancy if unopposed HRT is given

4.21 B C E p.38

    A the incidence is higher at the extremes of reproductive life

    C choriocarcinoma may present with brain metastases

    D partners are more likely to have different A and B blood groups

4.22 A B C D E p.35

4.23 C p.64; see also [12] p.341

    A HDL falls and VLDL rises

    B osteoporotic bone is normally calcified

    D 27% will die within a year of such a fracture

    E the only real contraindication to HRT is a history of a recent breast cancer

4.24 C p.57

    A the commonest cause is atrophic vaginitis/cervicitis

    B the contraceptive pill predisposes to ectropion formation

    D frank malignancy may be present when the smear is negative

    E carcinoma of the corpus uteri should always be excluded in this group

4.25 A B C D p.47

    E adrenogenital syndrome is associated with infertility

4.26 B C D p.4; see also [12] p.205

    A the frequency is 0.8%

    E PCOS is found in 82% of such cases

4.27 A D E p.24

    B they are often patent

    C the tubes are likely to be involved in an adjacent ovarian focus

4.28 **A B C E** p.50
   D sulphasalazine causes a decrease in semen count

4.29 **A** p.14
   B an IUCD interferes with the implantation of the blastocyst
   C the oral contraceptive pill is associated with a decrease in the incidence of endometrial malignancy
   D they inhibit the mid-cycle LH peak
   E progestogen-only pills do not inhibit lactation

4.30 **C D** p.109
   A brachytherapy is not used in this situation as the uterus has been removed
   B better results may be obtained from radical surgery
   E radiotherapy is recommended under these circumstances

4.31 **A D E** p.53
   B works at the level of the hypothalamus
   C multiple pregnancy rate is approximately 6%

4.32 **B E** pp.24, 136 and 138
   A it is usually a watery bloody vaginal loss
   C the aim is cytoreduction with surgery followed by chemotherapy
   D lichen sclerosus is not a premalignant condition

4.33 **A D E** p.98
   B koilocytotic cells characteristically have a perinuclear halo
   C a koilocytotic cell is one infected with HPV, not necessarily in the premalignant phase

4.34 **A B C D E** p.53

4.35 **B C D** p.26
   A such anomalies occur in 3–4% of the female population
   E only one pregnancy has been described in such cases, and the formation of a fistula is necessary to prevent haematometra, haematosalpinx, adenomyosis and endometriosis

4.36 **A E** p.129
   B secondary spread is common, particularly from adjacent organs
   C lymphatic spread from the fundus is to the para-aortic nodes
   D leiomyosarcomata arise in uterine fibroids

4.37 **A C D E** p.67
   B occurs in over 30% of these women

4.38 C D p.62
    A there are five stages in thelarche
    B precocious puberty is any menarche occurring at less than 8 years of age
    E there is an increase in the sensitivity of the threshold

4.39 B D p.91
    A around the third day
    C in the first week
    E rarely clinically apparent until the third day

4.40 A D p.70
    B pregnancy can occur afterwards although rarely
    C uterus can be retroverted
    E should be performed in the proliferative phase of the cycle

4.41 B E p.73
    A 500 000 follicles per ovary at menarche
    C the innermost structure is the polar body, followed by the zona
       pellucida, the corona radiata and the cumulus oophorus is the outermost
       structure of the four
    D the oocyte is arrested in meiotic prophase

4.42 E p.11
    A cervical cancer affects over 4000 women annually
    B HPV subtypes 16, 18 and 33
    C smoking and low social class are associated factors
    D peak incidence is in the fifth and sixth decades
    E proportionally more younger women have an adenocarcinoma

4.43 A B C D E p.76

4.44 A B D p.83
    C tetracyclines are contraindicated in children because of the dental and
       long bone effects
    E chemotherapy is the first line of treatment

4.45 A B D p.6
    C galactorrhoea occurs with hyperprolactinaemia of pituitary origin
    E the treatment is directed at the cause

4.46 A B C D E p.89

4.47 A B C p.106; see also [12] p.269
    D Doppler shift relates to the velocity of the red blood cells
    E no imaging is 100% correct

4.48 A B C E p.138
D there is a significant incidence of inguinal node metastases if the depth of invasion exceeds 1 mm

4.49 A B C D p.95
E associated with raised LH and a reversed LH/FSH ratio

4.50 B D E p.114; see also [12] p.843
A plateau precedes orgasm, resolution succeeds it
C male seminal fluids released prior to orgasm are rich in semen

4.51 A B C D p.81
E this is the treatment of epithelial cancer; combination chemotherapy is given for germ cell malignancy

4.52 A D E p.101
B there must be a 7 day symptom-free period in each cycle
C cause of symptoms unknown

4.53 B C See [12] p.23
A the clitoris has only two crura, the corpora cavernosa
D the vagina has no glands, such vaginal fluid being a transudate
E the incidence is 20%

4.54 C D E p.86
A chronic PID and tuberculosis
B acute PID is too painful to attempt intercourse

4.55 A B E p.19
C retroversion is not associated with ectopic pregnancy
D women over 35 are more likely to get ectopics

4.56 A B E See [12] p.23
C the nodes are medial, lateral and intermediate
D anastomoses mean that transection is not usually serious

4.57 C E p.109
A the SI unit is the Gray (Gy); 1 Gray = 100 Rads
B hypoxic cells are relatively radioresistant
D ionising radiation does not affect the metabolic function of the cell

4.58 B C D p.95
A progesterone only contraception does not prevent ovulation
E unaffected by diabetes

4.59 **A B C** p.95; see also [12] pp.81 and 125
   D serotonin will inhibit release
   E the ratio is 1:3

4.60 **C** p.59
   A 20–100 million per ml
   B 2–5 ml
   D less than 50% abnormal forms
   E a negative mixed agglutination reaction (a test for antisperm antibodies)

ANSWERS TO PAPER FIVE

The correct answers appear in bold
References refer to page numbers in *Key Topics in Obstetrics and Gynaecology* and references on p. 141 of this book

5.1 A B D p.1
  C ovaries are usually conserved in young women
  E only contraindicates if another risk factor is present

5.2 A B See [12] p.623
  C pelvic floor physiotherapy will improve symptoms in 50%
  D vaginal cones will improve 70%
  E any surgery for urinary incontinence may make detrusor instability worse

5.3 B D E p.135
  A vaginal carcinoma comprises 1–2% of female genital malignancies
  C the risk is for patients whose mothers took stilboestrol in pregnancy

5.4 A B C D p.3
  E not necessarily associated with uterine anomalies

5.5 B See [12] p.623
  A vaginal capacity and mobility must be assessed
  C morning residual, less than 200 ml and evening residual less than 150 ml
  D less than 5% will suffer from osteitis pubis
  E cystoscopy is always necessary

5.6 B C E p.117
  A a rash occurs with secondary syphilis
  D penicillin remains the drug of choice, e.g. Bicillin, a combination of procaine penicillin and benzylpenicillin

5.7 A C D p.3
  B frequency 0.8%
  E PCOS is more common in recurrent abortions

5.8 E p.16
>   A male sterilization is safer because it is less invasive and can easily be performed under local anaesthetic ·
>   B recanalization of the vas is of the order of 1–4:1000
>   C severe medical complications may dictate such a course
>   D the success is variable depending upon each case, but is usually of the order of less than 50%

5.9 B C E p.22
>   A retrograde menstruation is a commonly observed event, not always leading to endometriosis
>   D gestrinone is not a progestogen

5.10 A D E p.9
>   B the remnants of mesonephric origin are called Gartner's duct cysts
>   C Skene's duct cysts are periurethral cysts

5.11 A B D p.64
>   C HDL falls and VLDL rises
>   E such HRT will not reverse the osteoporosis

5.12 A B p.59
>   C oligospermia is defined as a sperm count of 10–20 million per ml
>   D results are poor
>   E this technique is used for sperm of low motility

5.13 B C D E p.17
>   A Bartholin's cyst will cause superficial dyspareunia

5.14 A D E p.73
>   B menstrual blood loss is 50% arterial, 25% venous and 25% capillary and diapedetic
>   C the basal arterioles appear uninfluenced

5.15 B C p.135
>   A distant spread of vaginal carcinoma is mainly via lymphatics
>   D sarcoma botryoides is a disease of childhood
>   E clear cell carcinoma occurs in young women whose mothers took diethylstilboestrol in pregnancy; the incidence should fall with cessation of this practice

5.16 A E p.19
>   B only 50% experience abnormal vaginal bleeding
>   C pain classically precedes bleeding but this is unproven
>   D vaginal ultrasound is the investigation of choice

5.17 **A B D** pp.71 and 107
 C the pelvis is relatively unaffected by respiratory motion
 E MRI may cause atrial fibrillation

5.18 **A B C E** p.98
 D both terms describe features of HPV infection; the latter suggests the presence of CIN

5.19 **B C D** p.29
 A diagnosis is often only made at laparotomy
 E the oral contraceptive pill can make fibroids grow

5.20 **C D** p.123; see also [14] p.141
 A cystometry calculates the intravesical pressure
 B detrusor pressure should be less than 15 cmH$_2$O
 E the bladder innervation level is S2–S4

5.21 **D E** p.129
 A the reverse is true
 B 20% of cases occur in premenopausal women
 C sarcomata are more likely to arise in a fibroid

5.22 **A B D E** p.32
 C a Boari flap is used when reimplantation is necessary

5.23 **A D** See [12] p.157 and [14] p.43
 B an absent cervix alone is very rare
 C the paramesonephric or Mullerian ducts form the tubes, uterus, cervix and upper vagina
 E 21-hydroxylase deficiency is the commonest cause

5.24 **A C** p.91
 B usually a small segment of lung collapses and is managed conservatively in the absence of risk factors, e.g. pre-existing pulmonary disease
 D unnecessary; the treatment of choice is local wound cleansing
 E small fistulae commonly respond to conservative measures, e.g. stenting of ureters or bladder catheterisation

5.25 **C D E** p.35
 A vault prolapse occurs in less than 2% of cases
 B 80% of patients complain of 'something coming down'

5.26 **A B C** See [12] p.3 and [6] pp.117 and 119
 D 45X or Turner's syndrome has an incidence of 1:2500
 E XXX females have increased height

5.27 A C D p.78

  B CA 125 (serum tumour marker) is often elevated in epithelial ovarian cancer

  E this programme is currently being evaluated

5.28 B D p.47

  A pituitary adenoma occurs in 40–50% of patients

  C drug of choice is bromocriptine

  E primary hypothyroidism occurs in 5% of cases

5.29 B E See [12] p.41 and [17]

  A the incidence is 1–2%

  C the amenorrhoea rate is 50%

  D endoscopic techniques are increasingly being used in malignancy

5.30 A B C D p.38

  E the figure is 42%

5.31 E p.50

  A day 21 progesterone should be over 30 nmol/l

  B D&C is seldom performed

  C PCT must be performed at mid-cycle

  D temperature charts show a 1°C rise at mid-cycle

5.32 A D See [12] p.377

  B the dose used is minimal

  C such a presentation is rare

  E there is no developed duct system and hence no lactation

5.33   p.11

  A HPV infection is associated with squamous cancer

  B proportionally more adenocarcinomata are found in younger women

  C this is a not infrequent event

  D the correct figure is around 20%

  E 85% of recurrences occur in the first 2 years

5.34 A B C E p.53

  D multiple pregnancy rate of up to 30%

5.35 A D See [12] p.219

  B it is best performed in the immediate preovulatory phase

  C it assesses sperm antibodies

  E the rate is 25%

5.36 **B D** p.138
  A the aetiology is unknown
  C the inflammatory infiltrate is subdermal
  E the rete ridges are elongated in hypertrophic dystrophy

5.37 **A C D E** p.53
  B cumulative success rate of 60% after 3 cycles

5.38 **B D** See [12] p.249
  A Kallman's syndrome is more common in boys
  C the ratio is greater than 17%
  E before the age of 16 years

5.39 **A C D** p.109
  B its use is unusual in ovarian cancer
  E the afterloading machine delivers a radioactive source into a mould, i.e. brachytherapy

5.40 **B C E** p.67
  A, D the definition of dysfunctional uterine bleeding means that all pathological causes have been ruled out

5.41 **A C E** See [12] p.269
  B 30–40%
  D non-absorbable sutures decrease the formation of adhesions

5.42 **D E** p.117
  A herpes simplex type 2
  B a DNA virus
  C treatment is more effective if commenced in the prodromal phase

5.43 **A B D** p.67
  C after medical treatment 20–40% of patients need further treatment
  E the use of a D&C is only diagnostic and not therapeutic

5.44 **B C E** See [12] p.279
  A the frequency is 1:10 000–16 000
  D it is a clue, but not diagnostic

5.45 **D** p.6
  A gonadotrophin levels are low
  B tunnel vision is associated with a pituitary tumour
  C these signs suggest Turner's syndrome
  E galactorrhoea results from excess prolactin secretion; prolactin is secreted from the anterior pituitary

5.46 **A B E** p.70

C operations can be performed in the proliferative phase of the cycle rather than after pretreatment with danazol

D submucous fibroids can be resected during the procedure

5.47 **C D E** See [12] p.291

A insertion can safely be done at 3–4 weeks postnatally

B Caesarean section carries no added risk

5.48 **A E** p.86

B bacteroides species are anaerobes

C not a proven pathogen; a common commensal

D beta-haemolytic streptococci are gram-positive cocci

5.49 **A B C** p.89

DE usually result in generalized abdominal pain and not pelvic pain

5.50 **A B E** See [12] pp.313 and 325

C 15% of PCOS women have hyperprolactinaemia

D virtually pure testosterone-secreting tumours can be seen in the presence of a normal urinary 17-ketosteroid excretion

5.51 **C D** p.81

A they are usually solid tumours

B Meig's syndrome occurs in association with a fibroma (benign)

E the role of chemotherapy is uncertain

5.52 **B C D E** p.95

A associated with a raised androstenedione

5.53 **A B C E** See [12] p.341

D oestrone is the major postmenopausal oestrogen

5.54 **C E** p.57

A the cervix should always be visualized to exclude an obvious carcinoma

B this situation warrants formal curettage under general anaesthesia

D this patient should be re-investigated to exclude dual pathology

5.55 **A B C D E** p.101

5.56 **A B C D** See [12] p.355

E 0.1% of sperm reach the Fallopian tubes

5.57 **C D E** p.38

A high-risk disease is treated with combination chemotherapy

B radiotherapy has no place in standard management regimens

5.58 **B C D** p.35

      A only occurs in multiparity

      E smoking does not in itself result in genital prolapse

5.59 **B D** See [12] pp.23, 413 and 519

      A the gonadal arteries arise from just below the renal arteries

      C USS is the imaging method of choice

      E CA 125 is useful but not definitive

5.60 **C E** p.11

      A these tumours have a relatively poor prognosis

      B cystoscopy is an essential part of the staging procedure

      D response rates are high; cure rates remain low

ANSWERS TO PAPER SIX

The correct answers appear in bold
References refer to page numbers in *Key Topics in Obstetrics and
Gynaecology* and references on p. 141 of this book

6.1 **A C E** p.3
    B family history does not appear to be important
    D *Candida* infection is not associated with abortions

6.2 **A E** See [12] p.653
    B an IVU is the best form of screening
    C augmentation 'clam' ileocystoplasty or caecocystoplasty
    D the majority of such lesions are idiopathic

6.3 **A C** p.64
    B oestrogen is superior to calcium in preventing osteoporosis regardless of
        bone density
    D there is an increase in facial hair
    E high HDL levels reduce the incidence of ischaemic heart disease; levels
        fall at the menopause

6.4 **A B** p.17
    C D E will all cause deep dyspareunia

6.5 **B C D E** See [12] pp.637, 665 and 667
    A more than once per night is abnormal

6.6 **C D** p.24
    A by definition a purulent infection leads to a pyosalpinx
    B drug therapy is the mainstay of treatment, surgery is rarely necessary
    E standard management includes platinum-based chemotherapy

6.7 **A B C D** p.19
    E risk of recurrence is over 15%

6.8 **A C** See [1] p.1330
    B it is the internal urethral orifice that forms the inferior boundary of the
        trigone
    D it is innervated by T11–L2 and S2–S4
    E the urethra is 4 cm long and 6 mm wide in the female

6.9 **A B C D E** p.129

6.10 **A D** p.29
   B   recurrence rate after myomectomy is as high as 30%
   C   not unless the fibroids become symptomatic
   E   vasopressin is often used to reduce blood loss at myomectomy

6.11 **B C D** See [12] p.385
   A   lichen sclerosus is not a premalignant condition
   E   HPV subtypes 6 and 11

6.12 **B C** p.98
   A   acetic acid is necessary to define characteristic features of CIN
   D   CIN commonly involves gland crypts
   E   laser treatment gives heat artefact which interferes with histological
       analysis

6.13 **B D E** p.32
   A   symptoms associated with a ureterovaginal fistula
   C   usually vaginal route is used for low vesicovaginal fistula

6.14 **C D E** p.126; see also [14] p.141
   A   up to 50% may be occasionally incontinent
   B   urodynamic evaluation is also necessary

6.15 **E** p.24
   A   tuberculosis is a rare cause of chronic PID
   B   caseation is typical of tuberculous salpingitis which does not exhibit
       features of acute inflammation
   C   adenocarcinoma is the commonest primary cancer
   D   surgery and cytotoxic chemotherapy are the main treatment modalities
       in primary tubal malignancy

6.16 **A C D E** p.35
   B   preoperative oestrogen is often used before surgery for procidentia

6.17 **A B D E** See [12] p.81
   C   they require 1% occupation

6.18 **B E** p.129
   A   the disease has a higher incidence in developed countries
   C   blood-borne metastases are rare and a late event
   D   high-grade tumours warrant adjuvant radiotherapy

6.19 **B D E** p.47
   A   gamma-aminobutyric acid release decreases prolactin release
   C   prolactin is secreted by the anterior pituitary gland

6.20 C D E See [12] pp.135 and 231
  A cyclofenil has no anti-oestrogen action
  B there is probably no difference

6.21 C D p.22
  A it is commoner in Caucasians
  B occasionally seen in the postmenopausal group
  E it is disputed that minimal endometriosis affects fertility

6.22 B C p.50
  A prolactin level over 800 mU/l is associated with anovulation
  D FSH/LH should be taken within the first 5 days of the cycle
  E submucous fibroids can result in implantation problems

6.23 A B C D E
  Re A [12] p.291 states 48 h, but Schering's Drug Data Profile [18] states
  72 h as being the upper limit

6.24 B C p.11
  A this is not a part of a standard radical hysterectomy and has been shown
    to be of limited clinical value
  D it is very unlikely that a previously irradiated patient will tolerate
    curative doses of radiotherapy
  E there is no proven survival advantage to chemotherapy, although the
    response rate is high

6.25 B C D E p.53
  A abortion rate increased by at least 10%

6.26 A B D E See [12] p.397
  C there is a 27% association with infertility

6.27 B D E p.117
  A yaws is caused by spirochaete bacterium
  C gonorrhoea is highly infective and commonly affects the rectum

6.28 B C E p.67
  A submucous fibroids are associated with menorrhagia
  D combined oral contraceptive pill is an effective form of treatment

6.29 B C E See [12] p.23
  A the sigmoid colon is posterior to the broad ligament
  D the rectum has no mesentery or appendices epiploicae

6.30 A B C D p.78
  E the aim of primary surgery is maximal debulking, with bowel resection
    a frequent requirement

6.31 **A B C E** p.70
     D most recent work agrees with this

6.32 **A B C E** See [12] p.581
     D urethral closure is passive and there is no known bladder neck sphincter

6.33 **A C** p.64
     B common sites of osteoporotic fractures are: neck of femur, vertebral body and wrist
     D there is no evidence that HRT with natural oestrogen increases the risk of thromboembolic disease
     E parenteral therapy avoids this effect

6.34 **A B D E** p.76
     C perforation should occur in less than 1% of cases

6.35 **B C D** See [12] p.615
     A PGs increase detrusor contractions
     E desmopressin (DDAVP) is useful in the non-hypertensive patient

6.36 **D** p.86
     A sexually transmitted disease is the commonest aetiological factor
     B laparoscopy is a useful investigation in suspected PID
     C an endocervical swab is preferred
     E pelvic clearance may be necessary; symptoms often persist after ovarian conservation

6.37 **B C E** p.89
     A only occurs in women of reproductive age
     D progestogens do not have long-term benefits

6.38 **A D E** See [12] pp.603 and 623
     B voiding greater than 7/day is frequency
     C 40% of such patients have significant anterior vaginal wall support

6.39 **A B C D E** p.38

6.40 **A D E** p.95
     B risk of endometrial cancer is increased
     C Metrodin is the drug of choice for ovulation induction

6.41 **B D E** See [13] p.231
     A the interval is 10 years
     C the rate of vertical transmission is 12.9%

6.42 B C p.138
A there are approximately 400 deaths in England and Wales per annum
D the peak incidence is in the seventh and eighth decades
E VIN is related to HPV infection; there is no association with lichen sclerosus, although these conditions may coexist

6.43 B C D E p.29
A menorrhagia only occurs with submucous fibroids

6.44 B C D E See [13] p.259
A mifepristone is a 19 nor-steroid

6.45 C D E p.59
A results after vasectomy are superior, particularly in the absence of antisperm antibodies
B the first sample has a high sperm concentration

6.46 A C D p.47
B E are not associated with hyperprolactinaemia

6.47 A C D E p.1; see also [13] p.317
B ureteric injury is more common at abdominal hysterectomy

6.48 A E p.78
B borderline tumours are of epithelial origin
C ovarian choriocarcinoma does not respond well to conventional treatment of gestational choriocarcinoma
D dermoid cysts are commoner in younger women

6.49 A B D E p.89
C retroverted uterus does not result in pain

6.50 B C D E See [14] p.55
A menorrhagia is menstrual blood loss greater than 80 ml per period

6.51 B C D p.135
A arises in the ovary
E arises in the ovary

6.52 A D E p.101
B not associated with PMS
C usually weight gain

6.53 A D See [14] p.157
B pain is the commonest presenting symptom
C clear cell adenocarcinoma has a poorer survival rate
E it is bilateral in 10–15% of cases

6.54 A C D See [12] p.81
> B they are less sensitive
> E AFP levels peak at 32 weeks

6.55 B D E p.95
> A LH is raised and there is a reversed LH:FSH ratio of 3:1
> C raised oestrone is associated with PCOS

6.56 B C E See [14] p.149
> A if a vaginal hysterectomy can be performed then it should be rather than a laparoscopic hysterectomy
> D laparoscopic hysterectomy can be performed for early endometrial carcinoma

6.57 A B See [12] p.397
> C black women have an increased incidence of fibroids
> D the incidence is decreased in cigarette smokers
> E HRT is not contraindicated

6.58 A C D See [12] p.55
> B light amplification by stimulated emission of radiation
> E thermal damage can happen to surrounding tissue

6.59 B C D E See [13] p.377
> A cervical cancer is the commonest indication

6.60 C D See [12] p.557
> A they do not inevitably proceed to malignancy
> B such tumours have relatively low levels of beta-hCG
> E the incidence is increased with increased maternal age

REFERENCES

1. Warwick R, Williams PL, eds. *Gray's Anatomy*, 35th edn. Harlow: Longman, 1973.
2. Turnbull AC, Chamberlain G, eds. *Obstetrics*. Edinburgh: Churchill Livingstone, 1989.
3. *Report on Confidential Enquiries into Maternal Deaths in the United Kingdom, 1988–1990*. London: HMSO, 1994.
4. *Bailliere's Clinical Obstetrics and Gynaecology*, Vol. 4, No. 2 (guest ed. Bygdeman M). Edinburgh: Churchill Livingstone, 1990.
5. *British National Formulary*, No. 26 (September 1993). London: BMA and RPSGB, 1993.
6. Brock DJH, Rodeck CH, Ferguson-Smith MA, eds. *Prenatal Diagnosis and Screening*. Edinburgh: Churchill Livingstone, 1992.
7. Whitfield CR, ed. *Dewhurst's Textbook of Obstetrics and Gynaecology for Postgraduates*, 4th edn. Oxford: Blackwell Scientific Publications, 1986.
8. Moore KL, ed. *The Developing Human, Clinically Oriented Embryology*, 2nd edn. Philadelphia: W B Saunders Company, 1977
9. *Review of Stillbirths and Neonatal Mortality in the Oxford Region*. Oxford: Oxford Regional Health Authority, 1992.
10. *Changing Childbirth. Part 1: Report of the Expert Maternity Group*. London: Department of Health, HMSO, 1993.
11. Spitz B *et al. American Journal of Obstetrics and Gynecology*, 1988; **159**: 1035–43.
12. Shaw RW, Soutter WP, Stanton SL, eds. *Gynaecology*. Edinburgh: Churchill Livingstone, 1992.
13. Studd J, ed. *Progress in Obstetrics & Gynaecology*, Vol. 10. Edinburgh: Churchill Livingstone, 1993.
14. Studd J, Jardine Brown C, eds. *The Yearbook of The Royal College of Obstetricians and Gynaecologists*. London: RCOG Press, 1993.
15. Sweet BR, *Mayes' Midwifery: a Textbook for Midwives*. London: Bailliere Tindall, 1988.
16. Craft TM, Upton PM. *Key Topics in Anaesthesia*. Oxford: BIOS Scientific Publishers, 1992.
17. Slade RJ *The Oxford five year review of TCRE*, unpublished data.
18. Schering PC 4 Drug Data. Schering Health Care Ltd, Burgess Hill, West Sussex. Product License Number 0053/0162.

COMPANION VOLUME
ALSO AVAILABLE FROM BIOS SCIENTIFIC PUBLISHERS LTD

Key Topics in Obstetrics and Gynaecology

R.J. Slade, E. Laird & G. Beynon
respectively University Hospital of Wales, Cardiff, UK; Northampton General
Hospital, UK; and Queen Elizabeth II Hospital, Gateshead, UK

A compact, easy-to-read text for trainee obstetricians and gynaecologists.
This book provides information on 100 major topics regarded as essential
knowledge to pass a postgraduate examination. Wherever possible, the
information is presented in a uniform, systematic format to encourage a
problem-based approach to clinical scenarios. The book is an ideal revision
aid with each key topic designed to be read at an individual sitting.

"Whilst one hesitates to recommend such volumes as a basis for learning,
this particular publication will be found by many to be a useful guide to
preparation for examinations from final MB to the MRCOG." -
Brit.J.Obstetrics & Gynaecology

Of interest to:

Trainee obstetricians and gynaecologists studying for a postgraduate
examination, such as the MRCOG part II; also general practitioners and
medical students.

Paperback; 296 pages; 1-872748-07-4; 1993

ALSO AVAILABLE FROM BIOS SCIENTIFIC PUBLISHERS LTD

Key Topics in Accident & Emergency Medicine

P. Howarth & R. Evans
respectively Royal Cornwall Hospital, Truro, UK; and Cardiff Royal Infirmary, UK

Provides the key information on acute injuries and sudden illness which commonly present at Accident and Emergency Departments. An ideal revision aid for postgraduate examinations and a useful source of reference for anyone who deals with acute problems, including paramedics, general practitioners and nurses.

Paperback; 1-872748-67-8; 1994;   332 pages

Key Topics in Anaesthesia

T.M. Craft & P.M. Upton
respectively Bristol Royal Infirmary, UK; and Radcliffe Infirmary, Oxford, UK

Essential information on 100 major subjects pertinent to modern clinical practice in anaesthesia. The uniform, systematic structure of the text is designed to encourage a problem-based approach to clinical scenarios. An ideal revision aid for trainee anaesthetists.

Paperback; 1-872748-90-2; 1992;   312 pages

Key Topics in Paediatrics

A.E.M. Davies & A.L. Billson
respectively Bristol Royal Hospital for Sick Children, UK; and University of Nottingham, UK

Describes important issues in child health, and the identification and management of problems. The information is presented in a systematic format which makes the book an ideal revision aid for a postgraduate qualification in paediatrics or child health.

Paperback; 1-872748-58-9; 1994;   348 pages

ORDERING DETAILS

Main address for orders

BIOS Scientific Publishers Ltd
St Thomas House, Becket Street,
Oxford OX1 1SJ, UK
Tel: +44 865 726286
Fax: +44 865 246823

Australia and New Zealand
DA Information Services
648 Whitehorse Road, Mitcham, Victoria 3132, Australia
Tel: (03) 873 4411
Fax: (03) 873 5679

India
Viva Books Private Ltd
4346/4C Ansari Road, New Delhi 110 002, India
Tel: 11 3283121
Fax: 11 3267224

Singapore and South East Asia
(Brunei, Hong Kong, Indonesia, Korea, Malaysia, the Philippines,
Singapore, Taiwan, and Thailand)
Toppan Company (S) PTE Ltd
38 Liu Fang Road, Jurong, Singapore 2262
Tel: (265) 6666
Fax: (261) 7875

USA and Canada
Books International Inc
PO Box 605, Herndon, VA 22070, USA
Tel: (703) 435 7064
Fax: (703) 689 0660

Payment can be made by cheque or credit card (Visa/Mastercard, quoting number
and expiry date). Alternatively, a *pro forma* invoice can be sent.

Prepaid orders must include £2.50/US$5.00 to cover postage and packing for one
item and £1.25/US$2.50 for each additional item.